Pharmacy Law Q&A Prep

Tennessee MPJE®

- ✓ **100 TENNESSEE LAW QUESTIONS**
- ✓ **100 FEDERAL LAW QUESTIONS**

PHARMACY TESTING SOLUTIONS

SECOND EDITION: REVISED FOR 2025

MPJE® is a registered trademark of the National Association of Boards of Pharmacy. This publication is neither affiliated with nor endorsed by the National Association of Boards of Pharmacy.

ISBN: 979-8-3747-8856-3

Table of Contents

Introduction

The Multistate Pharmacy Jurisprudence Examination (MPJE) is a pharmacy law exam developed by the National Association of Boards of Pharmacy (NABP). It assesses candidates' knowledge and competency in pharmacy law. The exam comprises 120 questions, combining federal and state-specific content, covering four content areas: Licensure/Personnel (22%); Pharmacist Practice (33%); Dispensing Requirements (24%); and Pharmacy Operations (21%).

This book is designed to help you prepare for both federal and state questions across all content areas. The first section presents 100 questions on federal pharmacy law, while the second section offers 100 questions on Tennessee state pharmacy law. An answer index with detailed explanations for each question is provided at the back of the book. When taking the MPJE, it's crucial to select the stricter law when discrepancies exist between federal and state regulations.

When preparing for the MPJE, focus fully, read each question carefully, and aim to simulate exam conditions by working through your practice questions without interruptions. The actual exam is 2.5 hours long, so it may be beneficial to time yourself during practice sessions to ensure you're allocating an appropriate amount of time to each question.

On the day of the exam, ensure you're well-rested, eat a substantial breakfast, and arrive at the testing center at least 30 minutes early for check-in procedures. Bring one valid, government-issued photo ID that includes a recognizable photograph and your signature, as this is required for admission to the testing center.

Good luck with the MPJE, and happy studying!

Federal MPJE Practice Questions

1. What was the first law requiring drugs to be proven safe before being marketed?
   a. Food, Drug, and Cosmetic Act
   b. Kefauver-Harris Amendment
   c. Pure Food and Drug Act
   d. Prescription Drug Marketing Act
   e. Durham-Humphrey Amendment

2. A pharmacist receives an urgent notification from a manufacturing company for a recall of a specific medication because it may cause serious adverse health issues or death. What type of drug recall is this?
   a. Class I
   b. Class II
   c. Class III
   d. Class IV
   e. Class V

3. What agency is responsible for the federal Controlled Substances Act (CSA)?
   a. Federal Bureau of Investigation (FBI)
   b. Food and Drug Administration (FDA)
   c. Department of Health and Human Services (HHS)
   d. Drug Enforcement Administration (DEA)
   e. United States Pharmacopeia (USP)

4. A pharmacist wants to know if generic warfarin tablets are bioequivalent to brand name Coumadin tablets. Where can this information be found?
    a. The Purple Book
    b. The Blue Book
    c. The Green Book
    d. The Orange Book
    e. The Red Book

5. Which of the following is NOT required on the manufacturer's drug container label for an oral drug product?
    a. Name of the manufacturer
    b. Expiration date
    c. Name of the drug or product
    d. Directions for administration
    e. Net quantity packaged

6. According to federal law, what age must the purchaser be to purchase a controlled substance without a prescription that contains opium?
    a. 16
    b. 18
    c. 21
    d. 25
    e. No age requirement

7. Which DEA form must be completed and submitted to the DEA upon discovering a theft or significant loss of controlled substances?
    a. DEA Form 106
    b. DEA Form 108
    c. DEA Form 222
    d. DEA Form 224
    e. DEA Form 363

8. Which of the following is a Schedule II controlled substance?
    a. Buprenorphine
    b. Butabarbital
    c. Mescaline
    d. Pentobarbital
    e. Modafinil

9. A non-preserved aqueous oral formulation that is compounded from commercially available drug products has a maximum beyond-use date (BUD) of _____ when refrigerated.
   a. 3 days
   b. 7 days
   c. 14 days
   d. 30 days
   e. 45 days

10. Practitioners who dispense methadone for detoxification must register for a narcotic treatment program using what form?
   a. DEA Form 222
   b. DEA Form 224
   c. DEA Form 363
   d. DEA Form 106
   e. DEA Form 41

11. Which FDA expedited review program is intended for drugs that treat serious conditions and fill an unmet medical need?
   a. Breakthrough therapy
   b. Instant approval
   c. Fast track
   d. Accelerated approval
   e. Priority review

12. Schedule II controlled substances CANNOT be transferred in which of the following scenarios?
   a. A pharmacy is closing and decides to transfer their Schedule II controlled substance inventory to another pharmacy
   b. A pharmacy is not renewing their DEA registration and therefore wants to transfer their remaining Schedule II controlled substances to another pharmacy
   c. A pharmacy ordered the wrong Schedule II controlled substances and wants to transfer them back to the supplier
   d. A researcher would like to transfer excess Schedule II controlled substances to a pharmacy to be dispensed to patients
   e. A pharmacy wants to transfer 2 bottles of Schedule II controlled substances to another pharmacy

13. A patient wants to refill a prescription but was not satisfied with the pharmacy that filled and dispensed the prescription the first time. The patient demands the prescription be returned so they can take it to a different pharmacy to obtain refills. The pharmacist should:
    a. Document the original fill information on the original prescription, keep a copy, and return the original prescription to the patient
    b. Offer to give a copy of the prescription to the patient, keep the original copy at the pharmacy, and recommend the patient request the prescription be transferred to another pharmacy if legal
    c. Void the original prescription before returning it to the patient and offer to transfer the rest verbally to another pharmacy
    d. Document the situation in the patient's profile and return the original prescription to the patient
    e. Inform the patient you can send the prescription by priority mail to the pharmacy of their choice

14. When a pharmacy submits a DEA Form 222 (single sheet) to purchase Schedule II controlled substances, who keeps the original copy of the DEA Form 222?
    a. The pharmacy
    b. The supplier
    c. The manufacturer
    d. The DEA
    e. The pharmacist

15. For which type of drug recall is there a possibility of temporary or medically reversible adverse effects, but the probability of serious adverse effects is remote?
    a. Class I
    b. Class II
    c. Class III
    d. Class A
    e. Class B

16. A drug has an NDC of 16103-0350-11. The 0350 represents:
    a. The manufacturer name
    b. The amount packaged
    c. The identity of the drug
    d. The location of manufacturing
    e. The route of administration

17. What set of regulations specifies the required minimum manufacturing standards for pharmaceutical products in the U.S.?
    a. Standards of Manufacturing Practice (SMP)
    b. Good Pharmaceutical Manufacturing Practice (GPMP)
    c. Requirements of Good Manufacturing Practice (RGMP)
    d. Regulations of Manufacturing Practice (RMP)
    e. Good Manufacturing Practice (GMP)

18. A prescriber may issue multiple prescriptions authorizing a patient to receive a total of up to a 90-day supply of a Schedule II controlled substance if certain conditions are met. Which of the following is NOT one of those conditions?
    a. Each separate prescription must be issued for a legitimate medical purpose
    b. The prescriber must include written instructions on each consecutive prescription indicating the earliest month in which a pharmacy may fill it
    c. The prescriber must conclude that providing the patient with multiple prescriptions will not create an undue risk of diversion or abuse
    d. The issuance of multiple prescriptions must be permissible under the applicable state law
    e. The prescriber must comply fully with all other applicable requirements

19. A prescription for lorazepam can be refilled a maximum of how many times within a six-month period?
    a. Zero
    b. Two
    c. Three
    d. Five
    e. Six

20. In order for buprenorphine to be prescribed, which of the following conditions must be met?
    a. The prescriber's liability insurance must provide buprenorphine indemnity
    b. The prescriber must have less than 30 patients to whom they prescribe buprenorphine
    c. The prescriber must have been granted a waiver from the DEA in order to prescribe buprenorphine
    d. The prescriber must have an active DEA license that includes the schedule in which buprenorphine is listed
    e. The prescriber must have an active "X" number

21. An example of an adulterated drug is:
    a. The name of the manufacturer is not included on the label
    b. A medication that has an unapproved color additive
    c. Active ingredients are missing from the bottle
    d. The drug causes an allergic reaction in the patient
    e. The drug container does not contain proper directions for nonprescription drugs

22. Which of the following is a mid-level practitioner?
    a. Physician
    b. Dentist
    c. Veterinarian
    d. Optometrist
    e. Podiatrist

23. Durable Medical Equipment (DME) must meet which standard(s)? Select ALL that apply.
    a. Can withstand repeated use
    b. Strictly for assistance with walking
    c. Limited to use for paraplegics
    d. Appropriate for use in the home
    e. Primarily for a medical purpose

24. What act regulates the sale and recordkeeping requirements for prescription drug samples?
    a. Prescription Drug Marketing Act
    b. Durham-Humphrey Amendment
    c. Pure Food and Drug Act
    d. Food, Drug and Cosmetic Act
    e. Kefauver-Harris Amendment

25. Which of the following can be determined from the National Drug Code (NDC) number on a medication bottle? Select ALL that apply.
    a. Manufacturer
    b. Specific drug
    c. Package
    d. Expiration date
    e. FDA approval status

26. Under the iPLEDGE Risk Evaluation and Mitigation Strategy (REMS) for isotretinoin, what is the maximum number of refills that may be authorized on a prescription?
    a. 0 refills
    b. 1 refill
    c. 2 refills
    d. 5 refills
    e. 11 refills

27. In which situation would it be illegal for a pharmacy to compound drugs?
    a. The quantity prepared is reasonable for filling existing and anticipated prescriptions
    b. Dosage forms are sold only to other pharmacies and not physician offices
    c. Ingredients in the compounded drugs meet national standards
    d. The compounded drug is not commercially available
    e. Interstate distribution of compounded drugs is no more than 5% of total prescriptions sold by the pharmacy per year

28. What DEA form is necessary to purchase or transfer Schedule II controlled substances?
    a. DEA Form 108
    b. DEA Form 222
    c. DEA Form 224
    d. DEA Form 225
    e. DEA Form 363

29. A patient calls the pharmacy and says they just got home from the hospital after having broken their leg. The patient cannot make it to the pharmacy to pick up their prescription for a Schedule II controlled substance that is ready to pick up. The patient asks if the pharmacy can mail the prescription to the house (mail delivery). How should the pharmacist respond?
    a. Controlled substance medications cannot be mailed
    b. Only Schedule III–V controlled substances can be mailed
    c. Controlled substances can only be mailed to the prescriber's office for office pickup
    d. The prescription can be sent to the patient through the mail
    e. The prescription can be sent to the patient as long as the drug name is listed on the package

30. Which of the following statements is/are true about narrow therapeutic index (NTI) drugs?

    I. Small differences in the dose or blood concentration may lead to adverse reactions

    II. They are not permitted to be prescribed

    III. They require careful titration or patient monitoring for safe and effective use

    a. I only
    b. II only
    c. I and III only
    d. II and III only
    e. I, II, and III

31. What act set the requirement for child-resistant closures for prescription drugs, non-prescription drugs, and hazardous household products?
    a. Poison Prevention Packaging Act
    b. Child Drug Safety Act
    c. Prevention of Hazardous Consumption Act
    d. Children Poison Prevention Act
    e. Hazardous Materials Safety Act

32. According to the Combat Methamphetamine Epidemic Act of 2005, the logbook requirement does NOT apply to individual single sales of packages of:
    a. No more than 60mg of pseudoephedrine
    b. No less than 60mg of pseudoephedrine
    c. No more than 50mg of pseudoephedrine
    d. No less than 50mg of pseudoephedrine
    e. All pseudoephedrine sales are required to be logged

33. Over-the-counter (OTC) drug advertising is regulated by the:
    a. Federal Trade Commission
    b. Food and Drug Administration
    c. Drug Quality and Security Commission
    d. Consumer Product Safety Commission
    e. None of the above

34. What information is required to be included in the transaction report transmitted from a manufacturer to a pharmacy when the pharmacy purchases bulk bottles of a medication?
    a. Transaction information, transaction history, transaction log
    b. Transaction purpose, transaction history, transaction ID number
    c. Transaction information, transaction history, transaction statement
    d. Transaction ID number, transaction code, transaction statement
    e. Transaction purpose, transaction history, transaction log

35. What law requires drugs to be proven effective (as well as safe) before being marketed?
    a. Durham-Humphrey Amendment
    b. Pure Food and Drug Act
    c. Prescription Drug Marketing Act
    d. Hatch-Waxman Amendment
    e. Kefauver-Harris Amendment

36. Which DEA registration form is used for pharmacies to register with the DEA to possess and dispense controlled substances?
    a. DEA Form 106
    b. DEA Form 222
    c. DEA Form 224
    d. DEA Form 225
    e. DEA Form 363

37. Re-importation of medications is only legal if performed by the:

    I.   Retail pharmacy

    II. Original manufacturer

    III. Wholesale distributor

    a. I only
    b. II only
    c. III only
    d. I and III only
    e. I, II, and III

38. Which of the following is true regarding the stocking and dispensing of methadone at retail pharmacies?
    a. Methadone may not be stocked or dispensed from a retail pharmacy; patients must obtain methadone from a narcotic treatment facility
    b. Methadone may be stocked at a retail pharmacy, but may only be dispensed as an analgesic
    c. Methadone may be stocked at a retail pharmacy, but may only be dispensed for narcotic dependence
    d. Methadone may be stocked at a retail pharmacy and may be dispensed as either an analgesic or for the short-term treatment of narcotic dependence
    e. Methadone may be stocked at any pharmacy and may be dispensed as either an analgesic or for the long-term treatment of narcotic dependence

39. What act requires health care facilities to report death or injuries caused by or suspected to have been caused by a medical device to the FDA or the manufacturer?
    a. FDA Modernization Act
    b. Medical Device Inspection Act
    c. Safe Medical Device Act
    d. Pure Food and Drug Act
    e. The Omnibus Budget Reconciliation Act

40. An example of a misbranded manufacturer's container of a drug would be:
    a. The drug causes an allergic reaction in the patient
    b. The container is made of a substance that leaches into the medication
    c. There is no quantity of the contents listed on the container
    d. The drug is exposed to unsanitary conditions
    e. The patient writes the indication for the medication on their prescription bottle

41. Which of the following requirements must be met for a controlled substance prescription to be valid? Select ALL that apply.
    a. Must be manually signed if it is a paper or faxed prescription
    b. Must be issued for a legitimate medical purpose
    c. Must be prescribed in the usual course of medical treatment
    d. Must be issued to an individual practitioner for the purpose of general dispensing to patients
    e. Must be dated and signed on the fill date

42. According to the FDA, a drug is considered to be an orphan drug if it is for rare diseases or conditions that impact fewer than how many people in the U.S.?
    a. 10
    b. 500
    c. 200,000
    d. 1,000,000
    e. 2,000,000

43. Which of the following ingredients has special labeling requirements if it is included in a product?
    a. Gelatin
    b. FD&C Yellow No. 5
    c. High fructose corn syrup
    d. Sorbitol
    e. Xanthan gum

44. In which case(s) is it appropriate to receive a faxed prescription for a Schedule II controlled substance?

    I. Patient is a resident of a long-term care facility (LTCF)

    II. Patient is enrolled in hospice program

    III. Medication is intended for home infusion therapy

    a. I only
    b. II only
    c. I and II
    d. II and III
    e. I, II, and III

45. What is the acronym of the voluntary reporting system for medication adverse events?
    a. VAERS
    b. FAERS
    c. ERSA
    d. MAERS
    e. AERS

46. Within how many days must a prescriber deliver a written prescription for a Schedule II controlled substance that was called in orally to be dispensed in an emergency situation?
    a. 3 days
    b. 5 days
    c. 7 days
    d. 14 days
    e. 15 days

47. A pharmacy intern wants to know where to find information on therapeutic equivalence between biologics. Which book contains this information?
    a. Red Book
    b. Purple Book
    c. Pink Book
    d. Orange Book
    e. Yellow Book

48. In which case(s) must an exact count be taken while performing a controlled substance inventory?

    I.   It is a Schedule II controlled substance

    II. The bottle holds more than 1000 tablets or capsules

    III. Containers are sealed or unopened

    a. I only
    b. II only
    c. I and II
    d. II and III
    e. I, II, and III

49. The scheduling of controlled substances at the federal level is performed by the:
    a. Food and Drug Administration
    b. U.S. Attorney General
    c. Drug Enforcement Agency
    d. National Board of Pharmacy
    e. Drug Enforcement Administration

50. A manufacturer of a prescription-only drug wants to reclassify the drug as an over-the-counter (OTC) drug. What is one of the forms that may be submitted to the FDA when requesting reclassification of a prescription-only drug to an over-the-counter drug?
    a. Emergency Investigational New Drug Application (EIND)
    b. Investigational New Drug Application (IND)
    c. New Drug Application (NDA)
    d. Abbreviated New Drug Application (ANDA)
    e. Marketed New Drug Application (MNDA)

51. You are a pharmacist that suspects a fake controlled substance prescription was called in to your pharmacy. You use the numbers in the provided DEA to verify if it is a true DEA number. It is indeed not a true DEA number because the last number is incorrect. The DEA number is BS5927683. What would be the correct last digit of the DEA number if it was accurate?
    a. 1
    b. 2
    c. 4
    d. 5
    e. 6

52. Which of the following prescriptions would likely be out of the scope of practice for a dentist?
    a. Tylenol #3
    b. Amoxicillin
    c. Lorazepam
    d. Atorvastatin
    e. None of the above; dentists are not limited to scope of practice

53. Who is authorized to sign a DEA Form 222 at a community pharmacy?
    a. Any pharmacist
    b. Any pharmacist or technician
    c. Only the pharmacist-in-charge
    d. Only the pharmacist who signed the most recent application for renewal of the pharmacy's DEA registration
    e. The pharmacist who signed the most recent application for renewal of the pharmacy's DEA registration or someone authorized under a power of attorney

54. What types of patients are included in a Phase I clinical trial for drug development?
    a. Large group of non-human animals
    b. Small group of healthy participants without the disease condition
    c. Small group of participants with the disease condition
    d. Large group of healthy participants without the disease condition
    e. Large group of participants with the disease condition

55. A pharmacy may keep which of the following records at a central location other than the location registered with the DEA?
    a. Controlled substance inventories
    b. Controlled substance prescriptions
    c. Controlled substance shipping and financial records
    d. Copies of executed DEA Form 222 orders
    e. None of the above may be kept at a central location; all must be kept at the pharmacy

56. Acetaminophen with codeine (Tylenol #3) is classified under which controlled substance schedule?
    a. Schedule I
    b. Schedule II
    c. Schedule III
    d. Schedule IV
    e. Schedule V

57. A patient is admitted to a hospital and does not remember the names of the medications that she takes at home. The hospital pharmacist calls the patient's outpatient pharmacy to obtain a list of medications. Which of the following statements is true?
    a. This is a HIPAA violation unless the patient has given signed consent for the information to be given to the hospital
    b. This is a HIPAA violation unless the patient has given verbal consent for the information to be given to the hospital
    c. This is a HIPAA violation unless the patient has given written and verbal consent for the information to be given to the hospital
    d. This is not a HIPAA violation because HIPAA does not apply to patients being treated in a hospital setting
    e. This is not a HIPAA violation because the information is being given to the hospital for treatment purposes

58. A warning stating "Caution: Federal law prohibits the transfer of this drug to any person other than the patient for whom it was prescribed" is required on the label on which of the following prescriptions?
    a. Schedule II controlled substances only
    b. Schedule II–IV controlled substances only
    c. Schedule II–V controlled substances only
    d. Schedule III–V controlled substances only
    e. All prescriptions require this warning under federal law

59. Registering with the FDA as an outsourcing facility allows a pharmacy to:
    a. Compound sterile products without receiving patient-specific prescriptions
    b. Act as a mail order pharmacy with the ability to send medications to multiple states
    c. Process prescriptions and medication orders remotely for another pharmacy, but not dispense any medications
    d. Repackage medications so that they can be used at hospitals and other institutions
    e. Order drug products listed on the FDA drug shortage list at a discounted cost

60. In the event of a breach of unsecured protected health information (PHI) at a retail pharmacy affecting approximately 900 patients, who must be notified? Select ALL that apply.
    a. All nearby pharmacies
    b. Prominent local media outlets
    c. Affected patients
    d. All patients who use the pharmacy
    e. U.S. Secretary of Health and Human Services (HHS)

61. Standards and requirements for preparing sterile compounded drugs to ensure patient benefit and reduce risks such as contamination, infection, or incorrect dosing are outlined in which of the following?
    a. USP Chapter <503A>
    b. USP Chapter <503B>
    c. USP Chapter <795>
    d. USP Chapter <797>
    e. USP Chapter <800>

62. Which of the following is/are required to register with the Drug Enforcement Administration (DEA)? Select ALL that apply.
    a. A patient who receives a prescription for a controlled substance
    b. A manufacturer that manufactures controlled substances
    c. A pharmacy that dispenses controlled substances
    d. A physician who prescribes controlled substances
    e. A pharmacist who dispenses controlled substances

63. Which of the following medications requires Risk Evaluation and Mitigation Strategy (REMS) monitoring?
    a. Hydromorphone (Dilaudid)
    b. Clozapine (Clozaril)
    c. Fluoxetine (Prozac)
    d. Zolpidem (Ambien)
    e. Metformin (Glucophage)

64. A DEA Form 41 is used to document which of the following?
    a. Purchasing of controlled substances from a manufacturer
    b. Transfer of controlled substances to a reverse distributor
    c. On-site destruction of controlled substances
    d. Significant loss or theft of controlled substances
    e. None of the above

65. What act set the requirement for tamper-evident packaging for some over-the-counter products in order to avoid risk of contamination?
    a. Safe Drug Packaging Act
    b. Federal Anti-Tampering Act
    c. Drug Contamination Prevention Act
    d. Federal Anti-Contamination Act
    e. Tamper-Evident Packaging Act

66. Drugs that have a high potential for abuse and severe potential for dependence with no currently accepted medical use in the U.S. are classified as:
    a. Schedule I
    b. Schedule II
    c. Schedule III
    d. Schedule IV
    e. None of the above

67. Which of the following is NOT required to be included on a manufacturer's container of an over-the-counter (OTC) medication?
    a. Warnings
    b. Inactive ingredients
    c. Poison Control Center phone number
    d. Purpose
    e. Directions

68. A nursing home patient who is prescribed an estrogen-containing product must be given a Patient Package Insert (PPI):
    a. Prior to the first administration only
    b. Prior to the first administration and every 30 days thereafter
    c. Prior to the first administration and every 60 days thereafter
    d. Only when requested by the patient
    e. None of the above

69. For how long is a DEA registration for possession of controlled substances valid?
    a. 12 months
    b. 24 months
    c. 36 months
    d. 48 months
    e. 60 months

70. Which of the following statements is/are true regarding DEA Form 222?

    I.   Executed copies of DEA Form 222 must be maintained separately from all other records.

    II. A defective DEA Form 222 may be corrected and reused.

    III. On the DEA Form 222, only 1 item may be entered on each numbered line.

    a. I only
    b. II only
    c. I and III only
    d. II and III only
    e. I, II, and III

71. An independent community pharmacy wants to start offering refill reminders to patients in the form of a postcard mailed to the patient's house. The fee for this service would be $2 per month. Which of the following is true regarding this service?
    a. This service cannot be provided because it creates a HIPAA violation
    b. Signed authorization would be required from each patient, as this is considered use of protected health information (PHI) for marketing purposes
    c. This service does not violate HIPAA, but patients cannot be charged a fee for refill reminders
    d. This service does not violate HIPAA, but the reminders must be transmitted electronically
    e. There are no barriers to offering this service and the pharmacy can proceed as planned

72. The expiration date on a bottle of metformin purchased from a manufacturer by a pharmacy is listed as 03/22. What is the expiration date of the drug?
    a. March 1, 2022
    b. March 19, 2022
    c. March 30, 2022
    d. March 31, 2022
    e. None of the above

73. A prospective drug utilization review (DUR) consists of reviewing all of the following aspects of a prescription EXCEPT for:
    a. Underutilization
    b. Therapeutic duplication
    c. Compliance with prescription labeling
    d. Appropriate dosing and regimen
    e. Drug interactions

74. Which of the following statements is required on an over-the-counter (OTC) package of acetaminophen tablets under the Federal Hazardous Substances Act?
    a. "Keep out of the reach of children"
    b. "Consult a doctor before use"
    c. "Do not use if pregnant or breastfeeding"
    d. "Prescription not required"
    e. "For adult use only"

75. A pharmacy dispenses and distributes a total of 50,000 doses of controlled substances in a 12-month period. How many doses is the pharmacy able to transfer to another pharmacy without registering as a distributor?
    a. 500 doses
    b. 1,000 doses
    c. 2,500 doses
    d. 5,000 doses
    e. 10,000 doses

76. The Occupational and Safety Health Administration (OSHA) requires that pharmacies do which of the following?
    a. Provide patients with information regarding the safe handling of hazardous medications
    b. Provide patients with Safety Data Sheets for hazardous medications
    c. Include the word "caution" or "warning" on labels for all hazardous medications
    d. Train all of their employees on the hazards of chemicals and on the protective measures they should take
    e. None of the above

77. The Poison Prevention Packaging Act (PPPA), which requires child-resistant containers for prescription and certain non-prescription drugs (with some exceptions), is administered by the:
    a. Food and Drug Administration
    b. Consumer Product Safety Commission
    c. Federal Trade Commission
    d. Centers for Medicare and Medicaid Services
    e. Occupational and Safety Health Administration

78. A pharmacy orders bulk bottles of ibuprofen and compounds ibuprofen suppositories. These suppositories are sold to other pharmacies that need to fill prescriptions but do not have the ability to make them. Which of the following terms best describes this practice?
    a. Compounding
    b. Dispensing
    c. Bulk compounding
    d. Manufacturing
    e. Outsourcing

79. Which of the following is true regarding the purchasing and selling of prescription drug samples?
    a. Drug samples may be purchased by a community pharmacy from a drug company and sold to patients at a standard price set by the FDA
    b. Drug samples may be purchased by a community pharmacy but must be given to patients free of charge
    c. Drug samples may only be given to a patient at a community pharmacy if the patient already has a prescription for the same medication
    d. Drug samples may be given to a pharmacy owned by a charitable organization and sold to patients at a reduced cost if the facility provides care to indigent or low-income patients
    e. Drug samples may be given to a pharmacy which is owned by a charitable organization that provides care to indigent or low-income patients, but must be given to patients free of charge

80. Which of the following is a valid method of ordering Schedule III medications from a supplier to restock a pharmacy's bulk medication supply?
    a. Mailing a hard copy of DEA Form 222 to the supplier
    b. Mailing a hard copy of DEA Form 224 to the supplier
    c. Faxing a copy of DEA Form 222 to the supplier
    d. Faxing a copy of DEA Form 224 to the supplier
    e. Sending an online order to the supplier with no additional form sent

81. Which of the following products is NOT required to be in tamper-evident packaging for retail sale?
    a. Acetaminophen tablets
    b. Children's diphenhydramine liquid
    c. Aspirin tablets
    d. Benzocaine/menthol lozenges
    e. Infant simethicone drops

82. A pharmacist may call a prescriber and receive verbal permission to change all of the following on a Schedule II prescription EXCEPT:
    a. Quantity
    b. Directions for use
    c. Drug name
    d. Drug strength
    e. Dosage form

83. A patient requests a copy of her prescription records from a community pharmacy. Within what time period must the pharmacy provide this information?
    a. 24 hours
    b. 3 days
    c. 7 days
    d. 10 days
    e. 30 days

84. Which of the following drugs has a REMS program due to a high frequency of birth defects?
    a. Lisinopril
    b. Thalidomide
    c. Zyprexa
    d. Atorvastatin
    e. Levothyroxine

85. Which law requires new drugs to be proven as safe and effective before approval?
    a. Poison Prevention Packaging Act
    b. Durham-Humphrey Amendment
    c. Kefauver-Harris Amendment
    d. Prescription Drug Marketing Act
    e. Drug Quality and Security Act

86. Anabolic steroids are classified under which controlled substance schedule under federal law?
    a. Schedule I
    b. Schedule II
    c. Schedule III
    d. Schedule IV
    e. Schedule V

87. Which act or amendment created the separation of drugs into two different categories, prescription (legend) and over-the-counter?
    a. Kefauver-Harris Amendment
    b. Omnibus Reconciliation Act
    c. Hatch-Waxman Amendment
    d. Durham-Humphrey Amendment
    e. Robinson-Patman Act

88. A patient picks up a prescription for Xarelto at a community pharmacy, but returns later in the day concerned that the prescription was filled with generic rivaroxaban. The pharmacist explains that the prescription was filled with the generic form of the medication because it was cheaper than using the brand name product. The patient asks if the generic will work as well as the brand name product. According to the pharmacist's drug reference, the two products have an FDA equivalency rating of AB. What is the proper interpretation of this code?
    a. The products are not bioequivalent, and the prescription should be filled only with brand name Xarelto
    b. The products have not been studied to determine bioequivalence, so a determination cannot be made
    c. The products have no known or suspected bioequivalence issues and are interchangeable
    d. The products may have actual or potential bioequivalence issues, but there is adequate evidence to use them interchangeably
    e. The code AB alone does not provide enough information to determine bioequivalence

89. DEA registration is NOT required for which of the following situations? Select ALL that apply.
    a. A nurse who is working in a physician's office where controlled substances are prescribed
    b. A pharmacist who regularly dispenses controlled substances at a community pharmacy
    c. A physician who occasionally prescribes controlled substances at a private clinic
    d. A patient who picks up a prescription for a newly prescribed controlled substance
    e. A pharmacy dispensing controlled substances

90. A drug manufacturer finds that bottles labeled "loratadine 10mg tablets" actually contain 5mg tablets, and issues a recall of the affected lot. Which of the following is true of this product?
    a. It is adulterated
    b. It is misbranded
    c. It is contaminated
    d. It is both adulterated and misbranded
    e. None of the above

91. A physician writes a prescription for ibuprofen 800mg tablets for a patient with rheumatoid arthritis. On the prescription, the physician adds a note that says, "please place this prescription and all future prescriptions in easy-open containers, as the patient is unable to open child-resistant bottles." Which of the following is true regarding this request?
    a. It is not valid because providers do not have the authority to request special packaging on a patient's behalf
    b. It is not valid because ibuprofen is not on the list of drugs exempt from the child-resistant packaging requirement under the Poison Prevention Packaging Act
    c. It is not valid because the provider must submit a separate signed form to make this request
    d. The ibuprofen can be dispensed in an easy-open container, but the blanket request to provide easy-open caps on all future prescriptions is not valid because only the patient can make such a request
    e. It is valid and a note should be made on the patient's profile to use easy-open containers on all prescriptions in the future

92. Which of the following would NOT be considered a potential part of a Risk Evaluation and Mitigation Strategy (REMS) program?
    a. Requiring special certification for pharmacies, practitioners, or health care settings that dispense a drug
    b. Requiring laboratory testing to ensure safe use of a drug
    c. Performing a financial assessment to ensure that a patient can afford a drug for the duration of treatment
    d. Providing a medication guide to patients which includes information about a drug
    e. Requiring that a patient enroll in a registry when they begin taking a drug

93. Retail containers of chewable low-dose 81mg aspirin (1.25 grain) must have special warnings for use in children including a warning regarding Reye's syndrome, and cannot contain more than:
    a. 10 tablets
    b. 30 tablets
    c. 36 tablets
    d. 48 tablets
    e. 60 tablets

94. Which of these is a valid DEA registration number for a mid-level practitioner?
    a. M11496023
    b. MT1200980
    c. CR5624112
    d. MM7411222
    e. BL115231

95. The FDA may require a medication guide be issued with certain prescriptions for which reason(s)? Select ALL that apply.
    a. When a drug has serious risks relative to benefits
    b. When patient adherence is crucial
    c. When the patient is a resident of a nursing home or other institution
    d. When drug information can prevent serious adverse effects
    e. When a pharmacist is unavailable to provide counseling on a new prescription

96. What act set the requirement that patients must be offered counseling on dispensed medications?
    a. OSHA 90
    b. DATA 90
    c. HCFA 90
    d. OPDP 90
    e. OBRA 90

97. Which of the following is/are NOT required to be packaged in a child-resistant container? Select ALL that apply.
    a. A container of 30 sublingual nitroglycerin tablets
    b. A methylprednisolone dose pack containing 21 tablets that are 4mg each
    c. A container of 100 aspirin tablets
    d. A prednisone dose pack containing 21 tablets that are 10mg each
    e. An albuterol inhaler

98. Prescription records must be kept for a minimum of _____ based on federal law.
    a. 1 year
    b. 2 years
    c. 3 years
    d. 4 years
    e. 5 years

99. A pharmacist dispenses a prescription for aripiprazole at an outpatient pharmacy. When is a medication guide required?
    a. Only for the first dispensing
    b. Every time the drug is filled, including refills
    c. Only if the patient requests
    d. The pharmacist may determine if a medication guide is necessary
    e. A medication guide is not required

100. To comply with Centers for Medicare and Medicaid Services (CMS) requirements, how often must a pharmacist conduct a drug regimen review for long-term care patients?
    a. At least once a week
    b. At least once a month
    c. At least once every 60 days
    d. At least once every 6 months
    e. Annually

Tennessee MPJE Practice Questions

1. A Tennessee pharmacy finds that a large quantity of controlled substance has been stolen after a break-in. What is the pharmacy obligated to do regarding the loss? Select ALL that apply.
    a. Close the pharmacy until all obligations are met
    b. Notify the Board of Pharmacy of the loss
    c. Submit a completed controlled substance inventory to the DEA
    d. Submit a copy of DEA form 106 to the Board of Pharmacy
    e. Submit a copy of DEA form 106 to the DEA

2. A patient is picking up a prescription for an eight (8) day supply of Lunesta at a pharmacy. The patient is unknown to the pharmacy staff and has forgotten all identification at home. Which of the following is true regarding picking up this prescription?
    a. Although the medication is a hypnotic, the patient does not need identification since it is less than a ten (10) day supply.
    b. The patient does not need identification to pick up this medication, regardless of its drug class, schedule or day supply.
    c. The patient must have identification since it is for a hypnotic and more than a seven (7) day supply.
    d. The patient must have identification to pick up any controlled substance.
    e. The patient must have identification to pick up any prescription, regardless of drug class schedule or day supply.

3. When is it permissible to have eight (8) technicians working under the supervision of one (1) pharmacist?

    I.   All technicians are certified

    II.   Two (2) of the technicians are certified

    III.   The board has granted permission to the pharmacy

    a. I only
    b. III only
    c. I and II
    d. I and III
    e. I, II, and III

4. A patient returns to a retail pharmacy three (3) months after having requested and receiving a partial fill of Ativan 1mg. The patient would like to fill the remainder of the prescription. What should the pharmacist do in this situation?
    a. The pharmacist can fill the remainder of the prescription since it has been less than six (6) months since the written date of the prescription.
    b. The pharmacist must contact the prescriber to ensure that the medication is still appropriate before filling the remainder of the prescription.
    c. The pharmacist must obtain a new prescription since the pharmacist is not permitted to dispense subsequent partial fills of a controlled substance prescription.
    d. The pharmacist must obtain a new prescription since the remainder of the prescription is void after a partial fill.
    e. The pharmacist must obtain a new prescription since the remainder of the prescription must be filled within sixty (60) days of the initial partial fill.

5. Which of the following services do not require a collaborative prescriber's diagnosis and patient-specific plan under a collaborative agreement with a pharmacy? Select ALL that apply.
    a. Buprenorphine treatment
    b. Influenza immunization
    c. Naloxone training
    d. Smoking cessation
    e. Treatment of lice

6. In which of the following situations would a faxed prescription from the physician's office to a retail pharmacy be allowed to serve as the original (i.e. no need to get an original hard copy of the prescription before dispensing)?

    I. Morphine prescribed for pain management for a patient under hospice care

    II. Norco prescribed for pain management for a terminally ill patient

    III. Oxycontin prescribed for end of life care for a long-term care facility resident

    a. I only
    b. III only
    c. I and II
    d. I and III
    e. I, II, and III

7. A thirty (30) year old female patient presents to the pharmacy with a prescription for chlordiazepoxide, once daily, #90. Which of the following is true for this prescription order? Select ALL that apply.
    a. Only a thirty-day supply or less may be dispensed of this prescription.
    b. The prescription can be refilled six (6) times after the initial fill if written by the prescriber.
    c. The prescription is valid for one (1) year from the date it was written.
    d. Valid identification is needed to pick up the prescription.
    e. The patient should have received counseling from the prescriber explaining the risk associated with using this drug during pregnancy.

8. A repackaged product dispensed to a patient in an institution must be labeled with pertinent information, including manufacturer name and lot number. When can the manufacturer name and lot number be omitted from the institutional label?
    a. A batch number is assigned to products prepared from the same manufacturer name and lot number and added to the label.
    b. The manufacturer name and lot number have not changed in ninety (90) days and are recorded, maintained and readily retrievable by the pharmacy.
    c. The products are intended for intravenous use.
    d. The products are loaded into an automated medication station (ex. Pyxis).
    e. The products are repackaged into unit dose packaging.

9. A patient has a prescription for Humulin 70/30 vial on file with the pharmacy. The patient does not have a prescription on file for syringes and would like to purchase them from the pharmacy. Which of the following is true when selling syringes to this patient?
    a. The pharmacy cannot sell the syringes to the patient as there is no proven medical need.
    b. The pharmacy may sell the syringes to the patient given there is a proven medical need.
    c. The pharmacy must call the prescriber to obtain permission to sell the syringes to the patient.
    d. The pharmacy must have permission from the Board of Pharmacy to supply syringes.
    e. The pharmacy must obtain a prescription for the syringes in order to sell them to the patient.

10. Which of the following statements is/are true concerning the automated dispensing devices used to dispense tablets and capsules?

    I. Drug lot numbers must be listed on the device.

    II. Drugs with different lot numbers can be mixed as long they are clearly labeled on the device.

    III. The device may only be loaded by a registered pharmacist.

    a. I only
    b. III only
    c. I and II only
    d. I and III only
    e. I, II, and III

11. Which of the following reference (electronic or printed) must be maintained at the pharmacy practice site?
    a. Good Manufacturing Practices
    b. Handbook of Drug Interactions
    c. State Pharmacy Laws
    d. The Orange Book
    e. The Purple Book

12. A patient has a prescription for Suboxone 12/3 mg, 2.5 films daily, #75, 2 refills. What is the practitioner's requirement when prescribing this dose to the patient? Select ALL that apply:
    a. Clearly document in the patient file the need for this higher dosage amount.
    b. Consult with an addiction specialist on dosing for the patient.
    c. Consult with a psychiatrist on dosing for this patient.
    d. The prescriber must be an addiction specialist to prescribe this dose.
    e. There are no prescriber requirements based on this dosage.

13. How long must a prescription order be kept on site at a pharmacy?
    a. 2 years from the date it was last dispensed
    b. 2 years from the date it was written
    c. 5 years from the date it was last dispensed
    d. 5 years from the date it was written
    e. Until all refills are used

14. Which of the following is true for continued education (CE) requirements for a licensed pharmacist?

    I. Continuing education is not required for pharmacists in residency.

    II. Fifteen (15) hours of continuing education must be live contact hours.

    III. Forty (40) hours of continuing education must be completed every (2) years.

    a. I only
    b. III only
    c. I and II
    d. I and III
    e. I, II, and III

15. What additional labeling is required for the <u>immediate container</u> of radioactive drugs? Select ALL that apply.
    a. The amount of radioactive material contained
    b. "Caution – Radioactive Material"
    c. The chemical form
    d. The radionuclide
    e. The standard radioactive symbol

16. Which of the following is a Schedule V controlled substance under Tennessee law?
    a. Alprazolam
    b. Carisoprodol
    c. Gabapentin
    d. Tramadol
    e. Zolpidem

17. Which of the following drugs can be issued from a satellite clinic within a federally qualified health center? Select ALL that apply.
    a. Atorvastatin
    b. Bupropion
    c. Clonazepam
    d. Hydrocodone-APAP
    e. Zetia

18. Which of the following patient identifiers would be permitted to substitute for a patient's social security number in the controlled substance monitoring database (CSMD) in the event a patient refuses to provide it to the dispensing pharmacy?

    I.   "999-99-9999"

    II. Patient's driver's license number

    III. Patient's telephone number

    a. I only
    b. III only
    c. I and II
    d. I and III
    e. I, II, and III

19. Which of the following drugs may be prescribed for assisting in patient weight loss? Select ALL that apply.
    a. Wegovy
    b. Dexedrine
    c. Phentermine
    d. Methylphenidate
    e. Saxenda

20. A patient has been receiving generic divalproex sodium DR 125 mg for epilepsy for the past six (6) months and has remained seizure free in that time. When filling this month's refill, the pharmacist notices the NDC number on the current bottle of divalproex sodium DR 125 mg is different from last month and the manufacturer has changed. What is the pharmacist obligated to do in this situation?

    I. Notify the patient or caregiver that the manufacturer has changed when picking up the medication.

    II. Notify the prescriber that the manufacturer is changing prior to dispensing the medication.

    III. Order the drug with the previous manufacturer to ensure continuity of treatment.

    a. I only
    b. III only
    c. I and II
    d. I and III
    e. I, II, and III

21. A home health patient has been issued a home care kit from a pharmacy. The home health provider had to remove sterile water for irrigation for emergency use. What is/are the pharmacy or provider obligation(s) in this situation?

    I. The pharmacy practice site must be notified of the opening and removal of drugs from the home care kit.

    II. The pharmacy practice site must restock and reseal the home care kit.

    III. The removal must be pursuant of a medical order or protocol and documented in the patient file.

    a. I only
    b. III only
    c. I and II
    d. I and III
    e. I, II, and III

22. Which of the following drug classes can only be dispensed in quantities equaling a thirty (30) day supply or less? Select ALL that apply.
    a. Barbiturates
    b. Benzodiazepines
    c. Hypnotics
    d. Opioids
    e. Amphetamines

23. Unused drugs are returned to an institutional pharmacy practice site. In which of the following cases could the drugs be kept without being destroyed?

    I.   Unit dose packaging

    II. Unopened, commercially prepackaged containers

    III. Unused prescription vial containing tablets

    a. I only
    b. III only
    c. I and II
    d. I and III
    e. I, II, and III

24. Which of the following is true regarding the use of tamper proof prescriptions in Tennessee?
    a. A prescription order written for inpatient use at a Tennessee hospital must be written on a tamper proof prescription.
    b. A unique serial number must be included on all tamper proof prescriptions for purposes of tracking the prescription.
    c. Out of state medical doctors must use tamper proof prescriptions when issuing directly to a patient or caregiver who intends on filling in a Tennessee pharmacy.
    d. Tennessee nurse practitioners must use tamper proof prescriptions when issuing directly to a patient or caregiver who intends on filling in a Tennessee pharmacy.
    e. Tennessee veterinarians must use tamper proof prescriptions when issuing directly to a patient or caregiver who intends on filling in a Tennessee pharmacy.

25. The prescriber must be notified when changing the manufacturer of which of the following drugs when the patient's disease has remained controlled with the same drug from a different manufacturer?
    a. Gabapentin for postherpetic neuralgia
    b. Lamotrigine for epilepsy
    c. Levothyroxine for hypothyroidism
    d. Primidone for essential tremors
    e. Valproic acid for migraine prophylaxis

26. Which of the following prescriptions could be dispensed to a patient in the event of the signing prescriber's death? Select ALL that apply.
    a. A new prescription order for a non-controlled drug within ninety (90) days of the date the prescriber died.
    b. A new prescription order for a non-controlled drug within one hundred eighty (180) days of the date the prescriber died.
    c. A refill for a controlled drug within one hundred eighty (180) days of the date the prescriber died.
    d. A refill for a controlled drug within ninety (90) days of the date the prescriber died.
    e. A refill for a non-controlled drug within one hundred eighty (180) days from the date the prescriber died.

27. Which of the following is true regarding the policy and procedure manual for sterile product compounding?

    I.   The manual must include procedures related to sanitation.

    II. The manual must include recommended attire for personnel engaged in compounding.

    III. Personnel engaging in sterile compounding must conduct an annual review on the policy and procedure manual.

    a. I only
    b. III only
    c. I and II
    d. I and III
    e. I, II, and III

28. Which of the following is true concerning the responsibilities of a pharmacist in charge (PIC)?
    a. Can only serve as PIC at two pharmacies or less
    b. Must conduct controlled drug inventory annually
    c. Must report to the Board any situation that causes serious injury or death
    d. Must work 50% of all hours in a pharmacy open one hundred (100) hours a week
    e. Responsible for staff pharmacist's non-compliance with state laws and regulations

29. A patient presents to the pharmacy to buy an over-the-counter cough and congestion product. The product contains dextromethorphan. Which of the following is true when buying this product?

    I.   The pharmacy may refrain from checking identification if the patient's outward appearance seems to be thirty (30) years of age.

    II. The pharmacy must check the patient's identification to ensure they are at least eighteen (18) years of age.

    III. The pharmacy may sell the product if the patient is less than eighteen (18) years of age with proof of emancipation.

    a. I only
    b. III only
    c. I and II
    d. I and III
    e. I, II, and III

30. In which of the following circumstances can a prescriber refrain from checking the controlled substance monitoring database (CSMD) before prescribing an opioid? Select ALL that apply.
    a. The patient is currently receiving hospice care.
    b. The opioid is prescribed for administration directly to a patient during the course of inpatient treatment in a hospital.
    c. The prescriber only intends on prescribing a 30-day supply.
    d. The prescription is for a 3-day treatment period with no refills.
    e. The prescription is for a 15-day treatment period with no refills.

31. What must a prescriber do prior to prescribing more than a three-day supply of an opioid or an opioid dosage that exceeds a total of a one hundred eighty (180) morphine milligram equivalent dose to a woman of childbearing age? Select ALL that apply.
    a. Advise the patient of the risk associated with opioid use during pregnancy.
    b. Consult with the patient's gynecologist about the appropriateness of the dose.
    c. Counsel the patient on appropriate and effective forms of birth control.
    d. Offer information about the availability of free or reduced cost birth control to the patient.
    e. Order and review a pregnancy test for the patient.

32. What quantity of prescription drug may a pharmacy practice site package to be dispensed for outpatient use from an emergency room?
    a. 12-hour supply
    b. 24-hour supply
    c. 48-hour supply
    d. 72-hour supply

33. Which of the following information is a minimum requirement for a prescription dispensing label from a retail pharmacy? Select ALL that apply.
    a. Pharmacy name, address and telephone number
    b. Prescription order serial number
    c. Prescriber telephone number
    d. Patient address
    e. Directions for use

34. What must a satellite pharmacy in a federally qualified health center do if there is a loss of video link with the central pharmacy?
    a. Cease all operation until the connection is reestablished.
    b. Cease all operation until the connection is reestablished and notify the Board of video link loss.
    c. Continue to prepare drugs for use, as video and audio link are encouraged but not required.
    d. Continue to prepare all drugs for use, given proper audio link is in working order.
    e. Continue to prepare non-controlled drugs for use, given proper audio link is in working order.

35. Which of the following practitioners may write a prescription for a drug with the purpose of causing or performing an abortion?

    I. Medical doctor

    II. Nurse practitioner

    III. Nurse practitioner with required training

    a. I only
    b. III only
    c. I and II
    d. I and III
    e. I, II, and III

36. A pharmacy is presented with a written prescription for atorvastatin 40mg, once daily, #90. The patient only wants to fill a thirty (30) day supply of the prescription due to cost. When initially dispensing this prescription order the pharmacist must record which of the following on the prescription order?

    I. The amount dispensed

    II. The date the prescription order was dispensed

    III. The signature of the dispensing pharmacist

    a. I only
    b. III only
    c. I and II
    d. I and III
    e. I, II, and III

37. How long is the term for an individual who is appointed to the Board?
    a. 4 years and maximum 1 full term
    b. 4 years and maximum 2 full terms
    c. 7 years and maximum 1 full term
    d. 7 years and maximum 2 full terms
    e. There are no term limits for Board appointees

38. Which of the following is a Schedule VI drug in Tennessee? Select ALL that apply.
    a. Marijuana
    b. Hemp
    c. Hemp derived cannabidiol (CBD)
    d. Tetrahydrocannabinol (THC)
    e. Synthetic cannabis

39. In which of the following situations may a prescriber use a written prescription for a Schedule II controlled substance? Select ALL that apply.
    a. The prescriber is a veterinarian.
    b. The prescriber issues sixty (60) or fewer prescriptions for Schedule II controlled substances annually.
    c. The prescriber issues the prescription pursuant of a patient-specific standing order.
    d. The prescription is issued with the intent of being dispensed by an out-of-state pharmacy.
    e. The prescription was issued during a technological failure.

40. What must be included in biannual controlled substance inventory?

    I.   The date of inventory

    II. The National Drug Code (NDC) and manufacturer of the drugs

    III. Whether the inventory was taken as of opening or closing of business

    a. I only
    b. III only
    c. I and II
    d. I and III
    e. I, II, and III

41. How often must a pharmacist renew their pharmacist's license?
    a. Every year
    b. Every two (2) years
    c. Every five (5) years
    d. Every ten (10) years
    e. License renewal is not necessary

42. A person taking possession of more than a seven (7) day supply of which of the following drug classes must present valid identification? Select ALL that apply.
   a. Barbiturates
   b. Benzodiazepines
   c. Hypnotics
   d. Muscle relaxants
   e. Opioids

43. If a prescriber is treating a patient with more than twenty (20) mg of buprenorphine daily for more than thirty (30) days what is the prescriber required to do?
   a. The prescriber is not permitted to prescribe this daily dose.
   b. The prescriber is not required to do anything further to prescribe this dose.
   c. The prescriber must be an addiction specialist.
   d. The prescriber must consult with an addiction specialist.
   e. The prescriber must make an effort to consult with an addiction specialist.

44. When can a Tennessee retail pharmacy accept a prescription order that was not written on a tamper proof prescription blank? Select ALL that apply.
   a. The prescriber is a medical doctor working outside of Tennessee.
   b. The prescriber is a nurse practitioner practicing under a Tennessee doctor.
   c. The prescriber is a veterinarian.
   d. The prescription order is for a patient in assisted living and was sent directly to the pharmacy.
   e. The prescription order was faxed to the pharmacy.

45. Who can request that a prescription for a controlled substance be partially filled?

   I.   The patient

   II. The prescriber

   III. The pharmacy benefit manager

   a. I only
   b. III only
   c. I and II
   d. I and III
   e. I, II, and III

46. Which of the following is true concerning a temporary absence of a pharmacist in a pharmacy? Select ALL that apply.
    a. Can only be two (2) hours daily
    b. Must display "pharmacist not on duty" sign
    c. Must be a physical barrier for prescription department
    d. Prescriptions may be sold from the will-call area
    e. Prescriptions may be compounded

47. Which of the following is required information that must be submitted to the Controlled Substance Monitoring Database (CSMD)? Select ALL that apply.
    a. Dispensing date of the controlled substance
    b. Estimated days' supply
    c. Patient identifier
    d. Source of payment
    e. Whether the prescription is new or a refill

48. Which of the following drugs can only be dispensed in quantities equaling a thirty (30) day supply or less? Select ALL that apply.
    a. Ambien
    b. Ativan
    c. Norco
    d. Ritalin
    e. Xtampza ER

49. A patient presents to a retail pharmacy to get a refill for metoprolol tartrate 50 mg, twice daily, #60. The prescription has 6 remaining refills. The pharmacist notices the signing prescriber for the prescription died 4 months prior to the date of fill. What is the pharmacist's option for refilling this prescription for the patient?
    a. The pharmacist can continue to refill the prescription for up to one-hundred eighty (180) days after the prescriber's death.
    b. The pharmacist must continue to refill the prescription for up to one-hundred eighty (180) days after the prescriber's death.
    c. The pharmacist can continue to refill the prescription until all refills have been used.
    d. The pharmacist must deny the refill since all prescriptions are void at the time of the prescriber's death.
    e. The pharmacist must deny the refill since it has been more than ninety (90) days since the prescriber's death.

50. Which of the following drugs have been approved by the Tennessee Board of Pharmacy for use in a home care kit? Select ALL that apply.
    a. Diphenhydramine
    b. Enoxaparin
    c. Epinephrine
    d. Naloxone
    e. Phytonadione

51. Which of the following is/are considered tamper resistant prescription features that meet federal Medicaid requirements?

    I.   One or more industry-recognized features designed to prevent unauthorized copying of a completed or blank prescription form.

    II. One or more industry-recognized features designed to prevent the erasure or modification of information written on the prescription pad by the prescriber.

    III. One or more industry-recognized features designed to prevent the use of counterfeit prescription forms.

    a. I only
    b. III only
    c. I and II
    d. I and III
    e. I, II, and III

52. A patient has asked for a copy of a previously dispensed prescription order in a retail pharmacy. What should the pharmacist do in this situation?
    a. The pharmacist can give the original prescription order to the patient as long as there is an electronic copy stored with the pharmacy software.
    b. The pharmacist can make a copy of the prescription order for the patient.
    c. The pharmacist can make a copy of the prescription order for the patient if the statement "Copy for Information Only" is written in black ink.
    d. The pharmacist can make a copy of the prescription order for the patient if the statement "Copy for Information Only" is written in red ink.
    e. The pharmacist cannot give a copy of the prescription order directly to the patient.

53. When must the indication for a drug be listed on the prescription label? Select ALL that apply.
    a. All prescription labels must include indication for a drug.
    b. The indication and diagnosis code are listed on the prescription.
    c. The patient requests that the indication be listed on the prescription label.
    d. The patient's caregiver requests that the indication be listed on the prescription label.
    e. The prescriber requests that the indication be listed on the prescription label.

54. A patient presents to a pharmacy to refill their prescription for clopidogrel 75 mg, once daily. The prescription has no refills remaining and the office is closed for the weekend. The pharmacist wants to ensure the patient does not miss doses while awaiting refill authorization. What can the pharmacist do?
    a. The pharmacist must await refill authorization since there is not a valid prescription on file.
    b. The pharmacist can fill a seventy-two (72) hour supply of the medication and await refill authorization.
    c. The pharmacist can fill a thirty (30) day supply of the medication and await refill authorization.
    d. The pharmacist can fill a twenty (20) day supply of the medication and await refill authorization.
    e. The pharmacist must obtain a new prescription order from a prescriber in an emergency room.

55. A patient presents to the pharmacy with a written prescription for Plavix 75mg, one every day, #30. The pharmacist dispenses the least expensive generic equivalent, clopidogrel 75mg, to the patient. What is the pharmacist's obligation when substituting a generic equivalent?
    a. The pharmacist may not make a generic substitution unless approved by the prescriber before dispensing.
    b. The pharmacist does not need to notify the patient that a generic equivalent has been substituted.
    c. The pharmacist must notify the patient of the substitution with a generic equivalent by a "face to face" interaction or phone call.
    d. The pharmacist must notify the patient of the substitution with a generic equivalent by noting the substitution on the prescription label.
    e. The pharmacist must notify the prescriber of the substitution with a generic equivalent by a facsimile or phone call.

56. A pharmacy outside of Tennessee would like to mail prescriptions to a patient residing in Tennessee. Which of the following is true for interstate prescription mailing requirements?
    a. A pharmacy outside of Tennessee cannot mail prescriptions to patients in Tennessee.
    b. A pharmacy outside of Tennessee can mail prescriptions to patients in Tennessee without any additional Tennessee licensure.
    c. A pharmacy outside of Tennessee must get Board approval to mail prescriptions prior to mailing prescriptions.
    d. A pharmacy outside of Tennessee must pay the same licensure fee required of a Tennessee pharmacy prior to mailing prescriptions.
    e. A pharmacy outside of Tennessee must pay an increased out-of-state licensure fee prior to mailing prescriptions.

57. A patient presents to a retail pharmacy with a handwritten prescription. The pharmacist is unable to read the prescriber's handwriting on the prescription. Which of the following is true concerning legibility of prescriptions? Select ALL that apply.
    a. A pharmacist may not dispense medication unless the prescription order is legible.
    b. A pharmacist must seek clarification for illegible prescription orders.
    c. A pharmacist can use their best guess based on legible parts of the illegible prescription order such as common drug strengths, indications and directions.
    d. A pharmacist is not liable for the delay caused by seeking clarification on an illegible prescription order.
    e. It is the duty of the prescriber to issue a legible prescription order to a patient.

58. A patient has requested a partial fill of their Belsomra prescription. The pharmacist must notify the prescriber of the partial fill of a controlled substance. Which of the following are/is (an) acceptable method(s) of notifying the prescriber in this case? Select ALL that apply.
    a. A notation in an interoperable electronic health record
    b. A notation in the patient's record maintained by the pharmacy that is accessible upon request
    c. A notation of "Partial Fill" on the prescription label dispensed to the patient
    d. Electronic or facsimile transmission
    e. Submission of information to the controlled substance database

59. What action(s) must a prescriber take when a female patient of childbearing age receives more than a three (3) day supply of an opioid that exceeds one hundred eighty (180) morphine milligram equivalent?

    I.   Counsel the patient on appropriate and effective forms of birth control

    II.   Advise the patient of the risks associated with opioid addiction

    III.   Advise the patient of the risks associated with opioid use during pregnancy

    a. I only
    b. III only
    c. I and II
    d. I and III
    e. I, II, and III

60. A pharmacy practice site that is a dispensing pharmacy must meet which of the following standards? Select ALL that apply.
    a. Consultation area that allows for sufficient privacy
    b. Drug stock may not be visible to the public
    c. Hot and cold running water
    d. Necessary counter and storage space
    e. Occupation of a space no less than three-hundred square feet

61. Which of the following must the Governor of Tennessee strive to ensure when making Board of Pharmacy appointments?

    I.   At least one serving member is a member of a racial minority

    II.   At least one serving member is over the age of sixty (60)

    III.   At least one serving member is a woman

    a. I only
    b. III only
    c. I and II
    d. I and III
    e. I, II, and III

62. Which of the following pharmacy personnel must wear appropriate identification showing name and title?

 I. Pharmacist

 II. Pharmacy intern

 III. Pharmacy technician

   a. I only
   b. III only
   c. I and II
   d. I and III
   e. I, II, and III

63. In which of the following cases must a pharmacist provide counseling to a patient or patient caregiver regarding a prescription order?

 I. An institution dispensing medication at discharge for outpatient use

 II. A long-term care facility administering drugs to inpatients

 III. A retail pharmacy dispensing a new prescription order

   a. I only
   b. III only
   c. I and II
   d. I and III
   e. I, II, and III

64. A pharmacist is responsible for a reasonable review of a patient's record prior to dispensing each prescription order. Which of the following must be evaluated when performing the review? Select ALL that apply.
   a. Clinical abuse and misuse
   b. Drug-allergy interaction
   c. Drug-drug interaction
   d. Efficacy of treatment option
   e. Under-utilization

65. Which of the following is true concerning pseudoephedrine base purchase limits? Select ALL that apply.
    a. A person may only purchase 5.6 grams in one (1) day.
    b. A person may only purchase 7.2 grams in thirty (30) days.
    c. A person may only purchase 43.2 grams in one (1) year.
    d. Limits apply to a prescription order from a prescriber.
    e. Limits apply to pharmacy generated prescription orders.

66. An electronic prescription is received by a retail pharmacy for Voltaren 75mg, one tablet twice daily, #60. The prescriber did not indicate that the brand name drug was medically necessary for the patient. What should the pharmacist do in this situation?
    a. The pharmacist, using their own discretion, may dispense any generic equivalent regardless of cost.
    b. The pharmacist must dispense the brand drug to the patient since it was written on the prescription.
    c. The pharmacist must dispense the least expensive generic equivalent in stock to the patient.
    d. The pharmacist must request permission from the patient prior to dispensing the least expensive generic equivalent in stock to the patient.
    e. The pharmacist must request permission from the prescriber prior to dispensing the least expensive generic equivalent in stock to the patient.

67. A pharmacist providing hormonal contraceptives to a non-specific patient as part of a collaborative pharmacy practice agreement with a prescriber must follow standardized procedures. Which of the following is/are required of the pharmacist pursuant of standardized procedure established by Tennessee? Select ALL that apply.
    a. The pharmacist must complete a risk assessment with each patient "face to face" to determine appropriateness.
    b. The pharmacist must complete a training program related to hormonal contraceptives.
    c. The pharmacist may dispense the hormonal contraceptive or refer the patient to a pharmacy that can dispense the hormonal contraceptive.
    d. The pharmacist must ensure that the patient has made a follow-up appointment with a primary care or women's healthcare provider.
    e. The pharmacist must provide a standardized fact sheet with indication, contraindication, method of drug use, importance of follow-up, and other information to the patient.

68. A patient has a new prescription order sent electronically to a pharmacy. The order is for lisinopril 10mg, once daily, #30, with 2 additional refills. The patient would like to fill the prescription for a ninety (90) day supply. What should the pharmacist do?

    a. The pharmacist cannot dispense a ninety (90) day supply given the drug class and controlled substance Schedule of the drug.
    b. The pharmacist cannot dispense a ninety (90) day supply since a new prescription order may only be filled for a thirty (30) day supply or less.
    c. The pharmacist can fill the prescription for a ninety (90) day supply without further action.
    d. The pharmacist must have the prescriber resend the electronic prescription order for a ninety (90) day supply.
    e. The pharmacist must obtain approval from the prescriber to dispense a ninety (90) day supply.

69. What is/are the requirement(s) for storing prescription order records?

    I. Each prescription order must be serially numbered

    II. Each prescription order must be filed sequentially by date filled

    III. Each prescription order must be stored at the pharmacy practice site for at least one (1) year after the last date dispensed

    a. I only
    b. III only
    c. I and II
    d. I and III
    e. I, II, and III

70. How much is the pharmacist in charge (PIC) required to work at the pharmacy practice site?
    a. 10% of hours the pharmacy is open
    b. 25% of hours the pharmacy is open
    c. 50% of hours the pharmacy is open
    d. 75% of hours the pharmacy is open
    e. There is no requirement for the PIC to be present at the pharmacy practice site

71. A patient comes into a retail pharmacy to buy over the counter pseudoephedrine. Who is permitted to counsel the patient and determine if the product is being used for a legitimate purpose? Select ALL that apply.
    a. A cashier
    b. A certified pharmacy technician
    c. A pharmacist
    d. A pharmacy intern
    e. A registered pharmacy technician

72. When is a pharmacist NOT required to counsel a patient when dispensing a prescription order in a retail pharmacy? Select ALL that apply.
    a. The patient or caregiver refuses counseling for a new prescription order.
    b. The patient or caregiver refuses counseling for a refilled prescription order.
    c. The pharmacist has deemed counseling for a new prescription order was not necessary and the patient or caregiver did not request counseling.
    d. The pharmacist has deemed counseling for a refill prescription order was necessary and the patient or caregiver did not request counseling.
    e. The pharmacist has deemed counseling for a refill prescription order was not necessary and the patient or caregiver did not request counseling.

73. Which of the following signs must be posted in all retail pharmacies?

    I. A statement that any person, regardless of age, who may be the victim of domestic violence may call the provided nationwide domestic violence hotline

    II. A statement that a teen involved in a relationship that includes dating violence may call a provided national toll-free hotline

    III. Contact information including the statewide toll-free number of the division of adult protective services, and the number for the local district attorney general's office

    a. I only
    b. III only
    c. I and II
    d. I and III
    e. I, II, and III

74. What must a pharmacist do to reinstate their license if it has been inactive for three (3) consecutive years? Select ALL that apply.
    a. Complete a period of pharmacy internship in Tennessee
    b. Provide written notice to the Board requesting an active license
    c. Satisfy all past due continuing education
    d. Successfully complete the NAPLEX
    e. Successfully complete the Tennessee jurisprudence exam

75. Which of the following medications would NOT require valid identification for picking up a 10-day supply at a retail pharmacy in Tennessee?
    a. Ambien
    b. Xanax
    c. Soma
    d. Ultram
    e. Vyvanse

76. In which of the following cases does policy allow a prescriber to issue a prescription?

    I.   Morphine for the prescriber for severe chronic pain

    II. Norco for a friend in a non-emergency situation

    III. Tramadol for the prescriber's own son in a true emergency

    a. I only
    b. III only
    c. I and II
    d. I and III
    e. I, II, and III

77. What are the requirements for the consumer member representing the public at large appointed to the Tennessee Board of Pharmacy? Select ALL that apply.
    a. Currently resides in Tennessee
    b. No financial interest in a health care facility or business
    c. No professional education as a healthcare provider
    d. Professional education as a healthcare provider
    e. Resident of Tennessee for five (5) years

78. Which of the following is/are exempt from registration as a pharmacy technician?

     I. A student enrolled in a formal pharmacy technician training program while performing experiential rotations

    II. Any individual performing tasks that may be performed by a pharmacy technician who is classified by the employer as a probationary employee

   III. Any individual performing tasks that may be performed by a pharmacy technician who is classified by the employer as a delivery driver

    a. I only
    b. III only
    c. I and II
    d. I and III
    e. I, II, and III

79. Which of the following is necessary for compounding cisplatin chemotherapy?
    a. Anteroom
    b. Bypass fume cabinet
    c. Horizontal flow cabinet
    d. Powder containment cabinet
    e. Vertical flow cabinet

80. What is the maximum number of technicians one (1) pharmacist may supervise?
    a. Six (6) technicians, and more if the additional technicians are certified
    b. Four (4) technicians, no matter certification
    c. Four (4) technicians, if two (2) are certified technicians
    d. There is no pharmacist to technician ratio in Tennessee
    e. Six (6) technicians, if three (3) are certified technicians

81. Which of the following drugs is/are required to be sent as an electronic prescription? Select ALL that apply.
    a. MS Contin
    b. Repatha
    c. Hydrocodone/APAP
    d. Librium
    e. Restoril

82. Which of the following is a Schedule V controlled substance in Tennessee? Select ALL that apply.
    a. Ativan
    b. Horizant
    c. Lomotil
    d. Lyrica
    e. Valium

83. Any licensed pharmacy that compounds sterile products must submit a report of high risk or batched sterile products to the Board every quarter. In which of the following circumstances is this quarterly reporting NOT required?
    a. Community pharmacy compounding for long term care
    b. Hospital pharmacy compounding for inpatient use
    c. Hospital pharmacy compounding for outpatient use
    d. Outsourcing facility compounding for hospice care
    e. Nuclear pharmacy compounding for clinic use

84. Who may have possession of keys to gain access to a retail pharmacy practice site? Select ALL that apply.
    a. Certified technician
    b. District manager
    c. Pharmacist in charge
    d. Staff pharmacist
    e. Store manager

85. Which of the following are requirements of pharmacists appointed to the Board?

    I.   Must be actively practicing as a pharmacist

    II. Must have been or is currently a preceptor

    III. Must have practiced pharmacy for a minimum of 5 years

    a. I only
    b. III only
    c. I and II
    d. I and III
    e. I, II, and III

86. Which of the following is required information that must be submitted to the Controlled Substance Monitoring Database (CSMD)? Select ALL that apply.
    a. Dispensing date of the controlled substance
    b. Estimated days' supply
    c. National Drugs Code (NDC) number
    d. Source of payment
    e. Whether the prescription is new or a refill

87. What registration(s) is/are required for a pharmacy to dispense controlled substances in the state of Tennessee?

    I.   DEA registration

    II. Board of Pharmacy registration

    III. Controlled Substance Monitoring Database (CSMD) registration

    a. I only
    b. III only
    c. I and II
    d. I and III
    e. I, II, and III

88. Which of the following may be omitted from the label of a sterile compound preparation for inpatient use?

    I.   Date of compounding

    II. Identification of pharmacist who prepared the compound

    III. Prescriber's name

    a. I only
    b. III only
    c. I and II
    d. I and III
    e. I, II, and III

89. Which of the following function must be personally performed by a pharmacist or pharmacy intern under the supervision of a pharmacist?
    a. Compounding of a prescription drug
    b. Making an offer to a patient for counseling
    c. Providing drug information to patients
    d. Receipt of an oral medication order
    e. Transfer copies of prescription order to another practice site

90. How often must a retail pharmacy submit information regarding dispensing of a controlled substance to the Controlled Substance Monitoring Database (CSMD)?
    a. Each business day but no later than the close of the following business day
    b. Immediately after dispensing the controlled substance
    c. It is recommended but not required for a pharmacist to submit information to CSMD
    d. No later than four (4) business days from dispensing the controlled substance
    e. No later than seven (7) business days from dispensing the controlled substance

91. In which of the following cases can a social security number for another person be used as the patient identifier when reporting to the controlled substance monitoring database (CSMD)? Select ALL that apply.
    a. The patient is a child who does not have a social security number and the social security number used is that of the parent or guardian.
    b. The patient is an animal and the social security number used is that of the animal owner.
    c. The patient is not available and the social security number used is that of the spouse.
    d. The patient is not available and the social security number used is that of the person picking up the prescription.
    e. The patient refuses to provide their social security number.

92. In which of the following cases is a prescription order for a buprenorphine monotherapy permitted? Select ALL that apply.
    a. Lower cost to the patient
    b. Patient is nursing
    c. Patient is pregnant
    d. Patient prefers monotherapy
    e. Prescriber prefers monotherapy

93. Which of the following must be true when substituting a generic equivalent drug?

    I.   The drug must be approved by the Food and Drug Administration (FDA).

    II.   There are actual or potential bioequivalence problems with the substituted drug that have been resolved with adequate in vivo or in vitro evidence supporting bioequivalence and is designated in the Orange Book as AB.

    III.   There are no known or suspected bioequivalence problems with substituted drug. Drug is designated in the Orange Book as AA, AN, AO, AP or AT.

    a. I only
    b. III only
    c. I and II
    d. I and III
    e. I, II, and III

94. What must be placed on the prescription label at the time of dispensing a compounded sterile product? Select ALL that apply.
    a. Auxiliary label
    b. Direction of use for outpatient preparations
    c. Expiration or Beyond Use Date (BUD)
    d. Name and amount of drug
    e. Pharmacy practice site name for inpatient and outpatient preparations

95. Which of the following is a controlled substance Schedule in Tennessee?

    I.   Schedule VI

    II.   Schedule VII

    III.   Schedule VIII

    a. I only
    b. III only
    c. I and II
    d. I and III
    e. I, II, and III

96. Which of the following are required to be licensed or registered with the Board? Select ALL that apply.
    a. Certified pharmacy technician
    b. Foreign graduate intern
    c. Pharmacist
    d. Pharmacy intern
    e. Pharmacy technician

97. A patient was given a seventy-two (72) hour supply of a medication that was out of refills. The patient returns to the pharmacy after the supply has been exhausted and is asking about the refill from the prescriber. The prescriber has yet to respond to the pharmacy's refill requests. What should the pharmacist do in this situation?
    a. The pharmacist must obtain a new prescription order from a prescriber in an emergency room or urgent care clinic for an additional emergency supply.
    b. The pharmacist must await refill authorization since the patient was already given a seventy-two (72) hour supply.
    c. The pharmacist can fill an additional seventy-two (72) hour supply of the medication and continue to await refill authorization.
    d. The pharmacist can fill a thirty (30) day supply of the medication and continue to await refill authorization.
    e. The pharmacist can fill a twenty (20) day supply of the medication and continue to await refill authorization.

98. In Tennessee, butyl nitrite is considered a controlled substance in which Schedule?
    a. Schedule I
    b. Schedule II
    c. Schedule V
    d. Schedule VI
    e. Schedule VII

99. What is the maximum amount of pseudoephedrine HCl 30 mg tablets (24.6 mg of pseudoephedrine base) a person may purchase over the counter every month?
    a. 234
    b. 240
    c. 292
    d. 300
    e. 365

100. Which of the following is true concerning the state-wide collaborative practice agreement for opioid antagonists?
   a. The agreement does not have to be maintained by the pharmacy.
   b. The pharmacist must have documentation of completion of an opioid antagonist training program within the previous two years.
   c. Opioid antagonists may only be dispensed to a person at risk of experiencing an opiate-related overdose.
   d. A pharmacist may only dispense an opioid antagonist pursuant to a patient-specific prescription drug order.
   e. A pharmacist may only dispense an opioid antagonist pursuant to a state-wide collaborative practice agreement.

Answer Index – Federal Questions

1 – a

The Food, Drug, and Cosmetic Act (FDCA) requires all new drugs to be proven safe for their labeled use before they can be marketed to patients. This act was passed in 1938 after a drug called elixir sulfanilamide caused mass poisonings and over a hundred deaths in the United States.

2 – a

Drug recalls are classified as Class I, II, or III, from most severe to least severe. A Class I recall is when a product may cause serious adverse health issues or death. A Class II recall is when a product has a low likelihood of causing serious adverse effects, but may cause some temporary or reversible adverse effects. A Class III recall is when a product is not likely to cause adverse health consequences.

3 – d

The Drug Enforcement Administration (DEA) is part of the U.S. Department of Justice and is responsible for the federal CSA. The Controlled Substances Act is available online on the DEA website. HIPAA is usually enforced by the Department of Health and Human Services.

4 – d

The Orange Book (the official title is "Approved Drug Products with Therapeutic Equivalence Evaluations") is the primary source for determining the therapeutic equivalency of drugs. The Purple Book lists biological products that are considered biosimilars and provides interchangeability evaluations for these products. The Red Book contains drug pricing information. The Green Book is for FDA-approved animal drugs.

5 – d

No directions for administration are necessary for oral drug products. However, if drugs are not for oral use, then the specific route(s) of administration must be stated.

Label requirements for the manufacturer container include: name and address of the manufacturer/packer/distributor, name of drug or product, net quantity packaged, weights of each active ingredient, route(s) of administration for non-oral medications, manufacturer control or lot number, expiration date, special storage instructions if applicable, and the federal legend (e.g. "Rx only").

6 – b

According to the DEA Pharmacist's Manual, a controlled substance listed in schedules II, III, IV, or V which is not a prescription drug as determined under the Federal Food, Drug, and Cosmetic Act may be dispensed by a pharmacist to a purchaser at retail, provided that:

- The dispensing is made only by a pharmacist and not by a non-pharmacist employee even if under the supervision of a pharmacist (although after the pharmacist has fulfilled his or her professional and legal responsibilities, the actual cash transaction, credit transaction, or delivery may be completed by a non-pharmacist)

- Not more than 240 cc. (8 ounces) of any such controlled substance containing opium, nor more than 120 cc. (4 ounces) of any other such controlled substance, nor more than 48 dosage units of any such controlled substance containing opium, nor more than 24 dosage units of any other such controlled substance, may be dispensed at retail to the same purchaser in any given 48-hour period

- The purchaser is at least 18 years of age

- The pharmacist requires every purchaser of a controlled substance not known to him to furnish suitable identification (including proof of age where appropriate)

- A bound record book is maintained by the pharmacist which contains the name and address of the purchaser, the name and quantity of the controlled substance purchased, the date of each purchase, and the name or initials of the pharmacist who dispensed the substance to the purchaser

- A prescription is not required for distribution or dispensing of the substance pursuant to any other federal, state or local law

- Central fill pharmacies may not dispense controlled substances at the retail level to a purchaser.

7 – a

A DEA Form 106, titled "Report of Theft or Loss of Controlled Substances," is a form that must be filled out and submitted to the DEA upon discovery of theft or significant loss of controlled substances. There is a section of the DEA Form 106 that allows the user to list out the controlled substances and quantities that were stolen or lost. Submitting a DEA Form 106 formally documents the situation and the pharmacy should retain a copy for their records. The DEA must also immediately be contacted by phone, fax, or brief written message to alert them of the situation. The local authorities should also be alerted.

There is no DEA Form 108. DEA Form 222 is for ordering Schedule II controlled substances. DEA Form 224 is for registration with the DEA. DEA Form 363 is for narcotic treatment facilities.

8 – d

Pentobarbital is a Schedule II controlled substance. It is a barbiturate. Schedule II controlled substances include but are not limited to: opiates and opioids, amphetamines and dextroamphetamine salts, pentobarbital, secobarbital, and phencyclidine. Mescaline is a Schedule I controlled substance. Butabarbital is a Schedule III controlled substance. Modafinil is a Schedule IV controlled substance. Finally, buprenorphine is a Schedule III controlled substance.

9 – c

A non-preserved aqueous oral formulation made from commercially available drug products has a maximum beyond-use date (BUD) of 14 days when refrigerated. Preserved aqueous formulations, such as topical and mucosal liquids or semisolid preparations, may have a BUD of up to 35 days, while non-aqueous dosage forms like capsules or powders have a BUD of up to 180 days.

The BUD must not exceed the expiration date of any ingredient used, and formulations with unstable components may require shorter BUDs.

10 – c

Here is a summary of DEA forms to know:

- DEA Form 222 is for ordering Schedule I or II controlled substances

- DEA Form 224 is for registering a new pharmacy

- DEA Form 363 is for new registration applications for narcotic treatment programs

- DEA Form 106 is for reporting loss

- DEA Form 41 is for drug destruction.

11 – c

The Food and Drug Administration has developed four distinct approaches to making certain types of new drugs available as rapidly as possible. The four approaches are:

- Fast track

- Breakthrough therapy

- Accelerated approval

- Priority review

Fast track is an expedited review process intended for drugs that treat serious conditions and fill an unmet medical need. Breakthrough therapy is a process designed to expedite the development and review of drugs which may demonstrate substantial improvement over available therapy. Accelerated approval is for drugs with long-term endpoints that are hard to measure during clinical trials, such as a decrease in mortality or increase in survival. These drugs are approved based on a surrogate endpoint. Finally, the priority review designation means the FDA's goal is to take action on the application within six months. "Instant approval" is not an FDA process.

12 - d

Schedule II controlled substances can be transferred in all of the given scenarios except for a researcher transferring Schedule II controlled substances to a pharmacy to be dispensed to patients. Researchers must be authorized to conduct research with Schedule II controlled substances. Researchers may transfer Schedule II controlled substances to another authorized researcher for the purpose of research. Researchers may not transfer Schedule II controlled substances to a pharmacy.

13 – b

Once a pharmacy has filled and dispensed a medication, the prescription is legally owned by the pharmacy and the original prescription can't be returned to the patient. However, it is acceptable to make a copy for the patient or the prescriber if needed. The prescription can be transferred to another pharmacy (if legal depending on the schedule and number of refills remaining), but the pharmacy that originally filled the prescription must retain the original copy.

14 - b

When purchasing Schedule II controlled substances, the pharmacy (purchaser) will fill out a DEA Form 222 and submit it to the supplier. The supplier receives the original form. The purchaser is required to make a copy of the original DEA Form 222 for their records. This copy can be retained in paper or electronic form. The purchaser does not have the option of keeping the original form.

15 – b
A Class II drug recall occurs when the product may cause temporary or medically reversible adverse effects, but the probability of serious adverse effects is remote.

16 – c
National Drug Codes (NDCs) are drug identification numbers that are unique to each drug manufactured. The NDC contains 3 sets of numbers:

1) The first set is either a 4- or 5-digit number and represents the manufacturer.

2) The second set is a 4-digit number that represents the identity of the drug.

3) The third set is a 2-digit number that is the product package size, such as the bottle count, blister packs, etc.

For example, we might have levothyroxine 50 mcg that is supplied as a 100-count bottle and a 500-count bottle from the same manufacturer. The NDC code will be the same except for the last 2 numbers because the bottle count sizes are different.

17 – e
Good Manufacturing Practice (GMP) is a set of regulations that determines minimum standards for pharmaceutical manufacturing in the U.S. The purpose of GMP is to uphold the safety and quality of drug products.

18 – b
According to the DEA Pharmacist's Manual, these are the criteria for an individual practitioner issuing multiple prescriptions for up to a 90-day supply of a Schedule II controlled substance:

- Each separate prescription is issued for a legitimate medical purpose by an individual practitioner acting in the usual course of professional practice

- The individual practitioner provides written instructions on each prescription (other than the first prescription, if the prescribing practitioner intends for that prescription to be filled immediately) indicating the earliest <u>date</u> on which a pharmacy may fill each prescription

- The individual practitioner concludes that providing the patient with multiple prescriptions in this manner does not create an undue risk of diversion or abuse

- The issuance of multiple prescriptions is permissible under the applicable state laws

- The individual practitioner complies fully with all other applicable federal requirements as well as any additional requirements under state law.

19 – d

Based on federal law, Schedule III and IV controlled substances can be refilled up to 5 times in a 6-month period from the date the prescription was written. Some states also apply this refill rule to Schedule V controlled substances. When a refill is dispensed for a Schedule III or IV substance, the dispensing pharmacist's initials, date the prescription was refilled, and amount of drug dispensed must be documented. Review page 49 of the 2022 version of the DEA Pharmacist's manual for information about the electronic record-keeping of Schedules III–IV refill information.

20 – d

Section 1262 of the Consolidated Appropriations Act of 2023 removes the federal requirement for practitioners to apply for a special waiver ("X" number) prior to prescribing buprenorphine for the treatment of opioid use disorder.

21 – b

Adulteration involves the integrity and composition of a product. If the composition or integrity of a drug is compromised, then the drug is considered adulterated. Some examples of adulteration include:

- A drug contains a decomposed substance

- A drug that is not manufactured under required manufacturing standards

- A drug that is stored in unsanitary conditions

- A substance of the drug container leaches into the drug itself

- A drug that is not pure or contains less than the listed amount of active ingredient

- A drug that contains an unapproved color additive.

22 – d

According to the Code of Federal Regulations, mid-level practitioners are defined as individual practitioners other than physicians, dentists, veterinarians, or podiatrists. Mid-level practitioners include but are not limited to: nurse practitioners, nurse midwives, nurse anesthetists, clinical nurse specialists, physician assistants, optometrists, homeopathic physicians, registered pharmacists, and certified chiropractors.

23 – a, d, e

DME is made for long-term use and must be able to withstand repeated use, be primarily for a medical purpose, and be appropriate for home use. It includes many different types of devices for individuals with a variety of conditions. Some examples of durable medical equipment include wheelchairs, crutches, canes, oxygen, ventilators, and hospital beds.

24 – a

The Prescription Drug Marketing Act (PDMA) of 1987 involves several laws regarding prescription drugs. Primarily, it regulates the storage, distribution, and resale of drug samples. It enforces recordkeeping requirements for prescription drug samples. The PDMA also prohibits hospitals and other health care entities from reselling their drugs to other businesses. This is because hospitals usually obtain drugs at a special rate. Finally, it regulates state licensing of wholesalers.

25 – a, b, c

An NDC number is a numeric, 3-segment code that identifies a drug by manufacturer (first 4 or 5 numbers), specific drug (next 4 numbers), and package (last 2 numbers). NDC numbers are unique to each drug and serve as a universal product identifier for drugs. The expiration date information is not included in the NDC number. By law, the FDA does not require that drug manufacturers include NDC numbers on labels, but it is highly recommended.

NDC numbers are published in an NDC Directory by the FDA. The labeler is responsible for the content of the NDC entry, not the FDA. Therefore, inclusion of information in the NDC directory doesn't mean that the FDA has verified the information. Additionally, assignment of an NDC number does not mean the drug has been approved by the FDA.

26 – a

Isotretinoin is an oral medication used to treat severe acne. Taking isotretinoin during pregnancy can cause birth defects, therefore this drug is highly regulated through a REMS program.

The REMS program for isotretinoin is called iPLEDGE. Under iPLEDGE:

- Only doctors registered with iPLEDGE may prescribe isotretinoin

- Only patients registered with iPLEDGE may receive isotretinoin

- Only pharmacies registered with iPLEDGE may dispense isotretinoin

- Patients may receive no more than a 30-day supply at a time

- No refills are allowed on prescriptions for isotretinoin

- Female patients who can get pregnant must use 2 separate methods of effective birth control 1 month before, while taking, and for 1 month after taking isotretinoin

- Female patients who can get pregnant must take a pregnancy test every month.

27 – b

Compounded drugs cannot be compounded, provided, or sold to other pharmacies or third parties. Compounded drugs cannot be commercially available, must meet national standards, must be a reasonable quantity for current or anticipated prescriptions, and distribution cannot be more than 5% of total prescriptions filled by the pharmacy per year. Drugs that have been removed from the market cannot be used in compounding.

Compounding may be an option to customize medications based upon a doctor's prescription. For example, compounding can customize a drug strength, remove an allergenic component, flavor a medication, and change the dosage form.

28 – b

A DEA Form 222 or an electronically equivalent program is necessary in order to purchase or transfer Schedule II controlled substances.

29 – d

The Schedule II controlled substance prescription can be mailed to the patient. Controlled substances used to not be able to be mailed, but this is no longer the case. The package must contain an inner package with the prescription and appropriate labeling, but must be placed in a plain outer container. The outside package cannot contain information about the contents of the package.

30 – c

Narrow therapeutic index drugs are drugs where small differences in the dose or blood concentration may lead to serious therapeutic failures or adverse reactions. These drugs require careful titration or patient monitoring for safe and effective use. They are permitted to be prescribed.

Some drugs with a narrow therapeutic index are: warfarin, levothyroxine, digoxin, lithium carbonate, phenytoin, and cyclosporine. Additionally, the FDA recommends that potency of the drug have a variability limit of 90% to 105% when the drugs are manufactured.

31 – a

The Poison Prevention Packaging Act (PPPA) set the requirement that prescription drugs, non-prescription drugs, and hazardous household products must have a child-resistant closure. The purpose was to protect children less than 5 years old from poisoning from accidental ingestion or exposure.

Patients may ask to not have safety caps on their medications, especially if they have conditions such as arthritis that make it difficult for them to open up the containers.

There are also several prescription drugs that are exempt from PPPA, such as nitroglycerin sublingual tablets, oral contraceptives in mnemonic dispenser packages, isosorbide dinitrate in sublingual and chewable forms, and more.

32 – a

The Combat Methamphetamine Epidemic Act of 2005 is a federal law that regulates "regulated sellers" including most pharmacies. It sets forth the requirements that these sellers must follow in order to sell ephedrine, pseudoephedrine, and phenylpropanolamine over the counter. Here are some requirements to know:

1) Products must be placed behind the counter or in locked cabinets

2) The identity of the purchasers must be verified, and a log of each sale must be obtained

3) The log must contain:
    - Purchaser's name
    - Address
    - Signature of the purchaser
    - Product sold
    - Quantity sold
    - Date
    - Time

4) The logbook must be kept for 2 years

5) All employees must be trained in the requirements and certify that they have received training

6) The quantity limits are 3.6 grams per day and 9 grams in a 30-day period. No more than 7.5 grams can be imported by mail

7) The logbook requirement does not apply to individual single sales packages of no more than 60 milligrams of pseudoephedrine

The DEA Pharmacist's Manual gives a complete list of proof-of-identity requirements.

33 – a

OTC drug advertising is regulated by the Federal Trade Commission (FTC). Prescription drug advertising is regulated by the Food and Drug Administration (FDA).

34 – c

Under the Drug Supply Chain Security Act, manufacturers are required to provide a transaction report (pedigree) for each product sold. Pharmacies are required to receive this information and pass it along if they further distribute the product. This allows the drugs to be tracked. The transaction report includes 3 parts, also known informally as the "3 T's": transaction information, transaction history, and transaction statement.

35 – e

The Kefauver-Harris Amendment requires that manufacturers provide proof of the effectiveness and safety of their drugs before these drugs can be approved. This was the first "proof-of-efficacy" requirement. The situation that prompted this amendment was the use of thalidomide in Europe that was marketed as a sedative-hypnotic drug that could be used during pregnancy, but it caused serious birth defects. Before the Kefauver-Harris Amendment, the Food, Drug, and Cosmetic Act (FDCA) of 1939 required drugs to be proven safe before being marketed.

36 – c

Pharmacies will use DEA Form 224 to register with the DEA to possess and dispense controlled substances. DEA Form 106 is to report theft or loss of controlled substances. DEA Form 222 to order and transfer Schedule I and II controlled substances. DEA Form 225 is used by manufacturers, distributors, importers, exporters, and researchers to register to conduct business with controlled substances. DEA Form 363 is used by narcotic treatment programs to register to conduct business with controlled substances.

37 – b

A drug product that is manufactured in the U.S., then exported to a foreign country, and then re-imported back to the U.S., is only legal if it is done by the original manufacturer. Re-importation is permitted by the original manufacturer if the purpose is for emergency medical care. Otherwise, re-importation of drugs is not permitted.

Some consumers want to engage in drug re-importation because drugs may be sold at a lower price outside of the United States. It would be a way to obtain access to these lower drug prices from countries such as Canada and Mexico, but it is illegal.

38 – b

Methadone is used for both the treatment of pain (i.e., as an analgesic) and in the detoxification and maintenance of narcotic addiction in patients registered in a narcotic treatment program. While a retail pharmacy may stock methadone, methadone can only be dispensed as an analgesic. Methadone can only be dispensed for the maintenance or detoxification of addicts when it is provided through a registered narcotic treatment center. It can be provided through one of these centers for either short-term detoxification (up to 30 days) or long-term detoxification (30–180 days).

39 – c

The Safe Medical Device Act (SMDA) of 1990 requires health care facilities to report death or injuries caused by or suspected to have been caused by a medical device to the FDA or the manufacturer. The goal is to quickly inform the FDA on the issue so the product can be tracked and potentially recalled for safety reasons. Some examples of medical devices that could be reported are: defibrillators, shunts, lab reagents, pulse oximeters, glucose meters, infusion pumps, wheelchairs, ventilator breathing circuits, needles, and catheters.

40 – c

Misbranding is inaccurate labeling on the drug container. If information is missing, inaccurate, or untrue, this is considered misbranding.

Examples of misbranding include: false or misleading information, unreadable material, omitting a medication guide, inadequate directions or warnings, omitting required information, etc.

41 – a, b, c

According to the Controlled Substances Act, a prescription for a controlled substance must:

1) Be dated and signed on the issue date

2) Include:
   - Patient's full name and address
   - Practitioner's full name, address and DEA number
   - Drug name
   - Drug strength
   - Dosage form
   - Quantity prescribed
   - Directions for use
   - Number of refills authorized
   - Manual signature of the practitioner

3) Be issued for a legitimate medical purpose by a practitioner acting in the usual course of professional practice

4) Not be issued in order for an individual practitioner to obtain a supply of controlled substances to keep on hand for the purpose of general dispensing to patients

Note: Even though the prescriber is responsible for ensuring that the controlled substance prescription is up to the lawful standard, a corresponding responsibility rests with the pharmacist who fills the prescription.

42 – c

A drug (or biologic) is considered to be an orphan drug if it is intended to treat a rare disease or condition that impacts fewer than 200,000 people in the U.S.

Sometimes, an orphan drug designation can be given to drugs citing a cost recovery provision, which is if the cost of research and development of the drug is not reasonably expected to be regained by sales of the drug.

43 – b

Several ingredients such as FD&C Yellow No. 5, aspartame, wintergreen oil, mineral oil, salicylates, sulfites, Ipecac syrup, and alcohol have special labeling requirements under federal regulations. FD&C Yellow No. 5, also called tartrazine, is a color additive that may cause an allergic reaction (itching and hives) in some people. Therefore, a product that contains FD&C Yellow No. 5 must identify so on the label.

44 – e

Normally, a faxed prescription for a Schedule II controlled substance cannot be accepted. However, there are 3 exceptions. Prescriptions for Schedule II controlled substances can be faxed and serve as the original prescription for patients residing in a long-term care facility, enrolled in hospice, or if the drug is to be compounded for direct administration by parenteral, intravenous, intramuscular, subcutaneous, or intraspinal infusion (which includes home infusion therapy).

45 – b

The FDA Adverse Event Reporting System (FAERS) is a database where adverse events from medications can be voluntarily reported. This provides post-marketing safety surveillance on medications.

Meanwhile, the VAERS stands for the Vaccine Adverse Event Reporting System, which is a national vaccine safety surveillance program run by the CDC and FDA.

ERSA, MAERS, and AERS are not drug-related reporting systems.

46 – c

A prescription for a Schedule II controlled substance can be called in orally to be dispensed in an emergency situation. The prescription should be immediately written down by the pharmacist. The quantity should only be enough to adequately cover the emergency period. The pharmacy needs to receive a hard copy prescription from the prescriber within 7 days after authorizing the emergency dispensing. This must also have the words "authorization for emergency dispensing" on the prescription and the date of the oral order written on the front. Prescriptions postmarked within the 7-day period are acceptable. If the prescription is not received in a timely manner, this should be reported to the DEA.

47 – b

The Purple Book contains information related to biological products and information regarding interchangeable biological products. The Orange Book provides information regarding therapeutic equivalence between drugs (excluding biologics). The Red Book is used for drug pricing and packaging information. The Pink Book contains information related to immunizations and vaccine-preventable diseases, as well as information on vaccine safety. Information and recommendation related to international travel (vaccines, diseases, information of other health risks) can be bound in the Yellow Book.

48 – e

An exact count must be made on controlled substances if they are Schedule I or II controlled substances, if they are controlled substances where the bottles contain more than 1000 tablets or capsules, and if the containers are sealed or unopened. Sealed or unopened containers do not need to be opened and counted, but the number marked as the container quantity must be used as an exact count.

49 – b

The U.S. Attorney General, as head of the Justice Department (which the Drug Enforcement Administration is under), may add, delete, or reschedule substances. A scientific and medical recommendation from the Food and Drug Administration is included in the decision.

50 – c

A full NDA must be submitted to the FDA when a manufacturer wants to request reclassification of a current prescription-only drug to be an over-the-counter drug. This is just one method of requesting reclassification, as there are four different methods. Another method is the FDA granting an exemption if determining prescription-only status is not necessary for the safety and protection of the public. A third method is filing a supplement to the original NDA (a "supplemental NDA") for review of the drug's safety and adverse events. The last method is if the Nonprescription Drug Advisory Committee recommends the ingredient contained in the drug be converted to a non-prescription status.

An ANDA is an application for the potential approval of a generic drug product. Both EIND and IND are applications regarding the development of a new drug. A marketed new drug application is not an existing type of application.

51 – a

In order to verify a DEA number, use the following process:

1) Add together the first, third, and fifth numbers.

2) Add together the second, fourth, and sixth numbers. Multiply this number by two.

3) Add the numbers together from steps 1 and 2. The last digit of the number you get from step 3 is the last number of the DEA number.

Using the DEA number BS5927683, the process would be:

1) $5 + 2 + 6 = 13$

2) $(9 + 7 + 8) \times 2 = (24) \times 2 = 48$

3) $13 + 48 = 61 \rightarrow$ Since the last digit is 1, the DEA should end in 1, not 3.

52 – d

Dentists must prescribe within their scope of practice. Accordingly, prescriptions written by a dentist must treat a disease of the mouth, treat discomfort of the mouth, or be used to facilitate a dental procedure. Atorvastatin is used to lower cholesterol. Other professions, such as optometrists and veterinarians, must also prescribe within their scope of practice.

53 – e

A DEA Form 222 must be signed and dated by the person authorized to sign the pharmacy's DEA registration. This means that only the pharmacist who signed the most recent application for renewal of the pharmacy's DEA registration may sign a DEA Form 222. Additionally, that pharmacist may authorize others to sign a DEA Form 222 by granting a power of attorney. A power of attorney must be signed by the registrant (the person granting the power), the person to whom the power of attorney is being granted, and two witnesses.

54 – b

Phase 1 clinical trials are conducted in a small group of healthy participants without the disease condition. Typically, the study size is around 20–80 people. The goal of the Phase 1 clinical trial is to study the properties of the drug and determine safety. Sometimes the Phase 1 clinical trial can include participants with the disease condition, but this is not as common.

Phase 2 clinical trials are conducted in a larger size group of 100 or more people, and these participants have the disease condition. Phase 2 clinical trials study the effectiveness of the drug.

Phase 3 clinical trials are conducted in a larger group of hundreds or thousands of participants who have the disease condition. The drug's safety, efficacy, and dosing are further studied. If a drug passes the Phase 3 study, then it can be approved by the FDA.

Finally, Phase 4 clinical trials are conducted after the drug is approved and looks at the safety and efficacy of the drug long-term, also called post-marketing surveillance.

55 – c

A pharmacy may keep shipping and financial data for controlled substances at a central location other than the registered location after notifying the nearest DEA Diversion Field Office. Executed DEA Form 222 orders, controlled substance prescriptions, and controlled substance inventories must be kept at the pharmacy location that is registered with the DEA and cannot be kept at a central location.

56 – c

Schedule III controlled substances have less potential for abuse than Schedule I or II drugs, and they have a currently accepted medical use in the U.S. Codeine by itself is classified under Schedule II, but in combination with acetaminophen it is a Schedule III drug.

57 – e

HIPAA permits the use of protected health information (PHI) for treatment purposes. Medical information can be shared to persons involved in the patient's care without written or verbal consent.

58 – b

The Federal Transfer Warning ("Caution: Federal law prohibits the transfer of this drug to any person other than the patient for whom it was prescribed") is required on the label of Schedule II–IV controlled substances when dispensed to a patient. Most pharmacies comply with this requirement by including this warning on all prescription labels. However, it is not legally required on prescription labels for Schedule V controlled substances and non-controlled prescriptions.

59 – a

Outsourcing facilities, also known as 503B facilities, are permitted to compound sterile products without receiving patient-specific prescriptions or medication orders. They are regulated by the FDA and subject to current good manufacturing practices. Compounded products must be distributed within a health care setting or dispensed directly to a patient or prescriber, and may not be sold or transferred to a wholesaler for redistribution.

A pharmacy that registers as an outsourcing facility would therefore be able to compound sterile products without receiving patient-specific prescriptions.

60 – b, c, e

The Health Information Technology for Economic and Clinical Health Act (HITECH Act) promotes health information technology to advance healthcare and the use of electronic health records. The HIPAA Breach Notification Rule is a part of this act.

It requires entities to notify affected individuals without unreasonable delay, and in no case later than 60 days following the discovery of a breach of unsecured protected health information. Breaches of 500 or more records also need to be reported to the Secretary of the U.S. Department of Health and Human Services (HHS) within 60 days of the discovery of the breach, and smaller breaches within 60 days of the end of the calendar year in which the breach occurred. In addition to reporting the breach to the HHS Secretary, a notice of a breach of 500 or more records must be provided to prominent media outlets serving the state or jurisdiction affected by the breach.

61 – d

The USP Chapter <797> describes the requirements of sterile compounded preparations, including responsibilities of compounding personnel, training, facilities, environmental monitoring, and storage and testing. USP Chapter <795> covers nonsterile compounding, and USP Chapter <800> describes safe handling of hazardous drugs. USP <503A> and USP <503B> do not exist as USP chapters; however, the terms 503A and 503B are used to designate compounding pharmacies.

62 – b, c, d

Every person or firm that manufactures, distributes, or dispenses any controlled substance must register with the DEA. However, patients who receive controlled substance prescriptions and pharmacists working in a pharmacy are exempt from DEA registration requirements. Therefore, pharmacists do not need to have a DEA number to dispense controlled substances.

63 – b

Clozapine is associated with severe neutropenia, which can lead to severe infections. Prescribers are required to be certified in the clozapine REMS program before prescribing clozapine. Pharmacies are also required to be certified in the clozapine REMS program to dispense clozapine.

64 – c

A DEA Form 41 is used to document the destruction of controlled substances. More commonly, a pharmacy will transfer controlled substances to an authorized reverse distributor for destruction. The reverse distributor then fills out DEA Form 41 to document the destruction of controlled substances.

65 – b

The Federal Anti-Tampering Act requires tamper-evident packaging of many over-the-counter products and cosmetics to avoid contamination issues and limit access. If the items were tampered with, it would be evident due to the packaging of these products. For example, some products have a tamper-evident closure cap, tamper-evident liner, and tamper-evident tape. The act was passed in response to the Tylenol poisoning deaths in Chicago in 1982, where the Tylenol capsules were contaminated with cyanide.

66 – a

Schedule I controlled substances include drugs that have a high potential for abuse and severe potential for dependence, with no currently accepted medical use in the U.S. This includes heroin, lysergic acid diethylamide (LSD), mescaline, and methaqualone, among others.

67 – c

Manufacturer's containers of OTC medications are required to display the following information: identity of the product (active ingredient), inactive ingredient(s), purpose, use(s), warnings, directions, and storage information.

Other information that is not required, but may be included, is as follows: net quantity of contents, name and address of the manufacturer/packager/distributor, lot number or batch code, expiration date, and instructions for what to do if an overdose occurs.

While the Poison Control Center phone number is included on some OTC medications, it is not required by federal law.

68 – b

Patient Package Inserts (PPIs) must be provided to patients in acute-care hospitals or long-term care facilities prior to the first administration and every 30 days thereafter. They are required for oral contraceptives and estrogen-containing products.

69 – c

DEA registration permits pharmacies, manufacturers, distributors, importers, exporters, and researchers to possess controlled substances. A DEA registration is valid for 36 months. Registrants will receive renewal notification approximately 60 days prior to the DEA registration expiration date.

70 – c

For recordkeeping requirements, executed copies of DEA Form 222 must be maintained separately from all other records. If a pharmacy stores these forms electronically, then the electronic records are deemed separate if such copies are readily retrievable from all other electronic records. A defective DEA Form 222 cannot be corrected and needs to be replaced by a new form. Finally, when filling out the DEA Form 222, only 1 item may be entered on each numbered line.

71 – e

Under the Health Insurance Portability and Accountability Act (HIPAA) Privacy Rule, a communication is not considered "marketing" if it is made for the treatment of the individual. Therefore, refill reminders for currently prescribed medications (or one that has not lapsed for more than 90 days) are not considered marketing. Therefore, offering this service is not a HIPAA violation. Patients may be charged for this service as long as any payment made to the pharmacy is reasonable and related to the pharmacy's cost of making the communication. Mailed refill reminders are valid, as well as electronic refill reminders.

As a note, the HIPAA Privacy Rule defines marketing as making "a communication about a product or service that encourages recipients of the communication to purchase or use the product or service." An entity would need to receive authorization from the patient to send out marketing communications.

72 – d

Manufacturer's expiration dates may be expressed as a day, month, and year, or as just a month and year. If it is written as only month and year, the drug expires on the last day of the listed month. The drug is safe to use on the expiration date, but not after.

73 – c

A prospective DUR consists of reviewing a prescription for adverse effects, therapeutic duplication, drug-disease interactions and contraindications, drug dosing and regimen, drug allergies, clinical misuse or abuse, drug interactions, medication appropriateness, overutilization, underutilization, and pregnancy alerts. Ensuring compliance with prescription labeling is not part of the prospective DUR.

74 – a

The purpose of the Federal Hazardous Substances Act (FHSA) is to protect consumers from hazardous or toxic substances. The FHSA requires precautionary labeling on the immediate container of hazardous household products, which includes certain OTC medications. Medication packages would include the statement, "Keep out of the reach of children." Depending on the hazardous substance, additional warnings and statements, such as "handle with gloves" or "harmful if swallowed," may be required. The warning "Keep out of the reach of children" applies to OTC drugs and not FDA-regulated drugs.

75 – c

The 5% rule states that a pharmacy does not have to register with the DEA as a distributor if the total quantity of controlled substances distributed during a 12-month period does not exceed 5% of the total quantity of all controlled substances dispensed and distributed during that period.

76 – d

The Occupational and Safety Health Administration (OSHA) requires that employers meet the Hazardous Communication Standard. This includes having a Hazardous Communication Plan, which lists hazardous chemicals in the workplace, and ensuring that all such products are appropriately labeled and have a Safety Data Sheet. Workers must be trained on the hazards of chemicals, appropriate protective measures, and where to find more information. The purpose of OSHA is to protect employees, which is separate from laws intended to protect consumers and patients.

77 – b

The Consumer Product Safety Commission administers the Poison Prevention Packaging Act (PPPA). This act requires child-resistant containers for all prescriptions and certain non-prescription drugs, unless there is an exemption for a specific drug or circumstance.

78 – d

Bulk compounding of products in order to sell them to other pharmacies is considered "manufacturing," which is regulated by the FDA. Note that for manufacturing, a patient-specific prescription is not required. So, in this case, since there is not a patient-specific prescription involved, the mass production of ibuprofen suppositories is considered manufacturing. On the other hand, "compounding" is typically regulated by state boards of pharmacy and is limited to compounding prescriptions for individual patients pursuant to a prescription.

79 – e

The Prescription Drug Marketing Act bans most pharmacies from purchasing, trading, selling, or possessing prescription drug samples. The only exception is for pharmacies that are owned by a charitable organization or by a city, state, or county government and that are part of a health care entity providing care to indigent or low-income patients at no or reduced cost. In this case, samples may only be provided at no cost to the patients.

80 – e

DEA Form 222 is used to transfer and order Schedule II controlled substances. The DEA used to allow this form to be faxed, but not anymore. A DEA Form 224 is needed for a pharmacy to dispense controlled substances. Schedule III–V controlled substances may be ordered through normal ordering processes from wholesalers or manufacturers, but must be documented by the pharmacy with an invoice upon receipt. The common term used for ordering Schedule III–V controlled substances is "using an invoice."

81 – d

Manufacturers and packagers of over-the-counter drugs for sale at retail must package products in tamper-evident packaging, with some exceptions. The exceptions are dermatological, dentifrice, insulin, or lozenge products.

82 – c

A pharmacist may not change the following items on a Schedule II controlled substance prescription: name of the patient, name of the drug, and name of the prescriber. All other information, including quantity, directions for use, drug strength, and dosage form, may be changed with the verbal permission of the prescriber as long as the change is documented on the prescription.

83 – e

Patients have a right to obtain a copy of their protected health information. Pharmacies must comply with such a request within 30 days. If there is a delay, the patient must be notified of the reason for delay and the pharmacy may extend the time by no more than 30 additional days. Normally, pharmacies are able to give a copy of the prescription record on the day of the request.

84 - b

Thalidomide is an immunomodulatory agent as well as a chemotherapy drug. Thalidomide causes a high frequency of birth defects in pregnant females. Babies were born with missing or deformed arms and legs. Therefore, the REMS program was developed to ensure safe use and monitoring of thalidomide.

85 – c

The Kefauver-Harris Amendment of 1962 is more commonly known as the "Drug Efficacy Amendment." It requires new drugs to be proven as safe and effective before they are approved. It also allows the FDA to establish good drug manufacturing practices and gives the FDA jurisdiction over prescription drug advertising, which must include accurate information about side effects. It also controls the marketing of generic drugs to keep them from being sold as expensive medications under new trade names.

86 – c

Anabolic steroids are classified as Schedule III controlled substances under federal law. An example of an anabolic steroid is testosterone.

87 – d

The Durham-Humphrey Amendment created two separate categories of drugs, prescription (legend) and over-the-counter (OTC). Prescription drugs require a prescription and must be dispensed under medical supervision. OTC drugs can be obtained without a prescription and do not require medical supervision.

88 – d

Generic bioequivalence information is found in the FDA Orange Book. A two-letter coding system indicates equivalency, with the first letter being key. Codes that start with the letter A indicate that the FDA considers the drug products to be pharmaceutically and therapeutically equivalent. Codes that start with the letter B indicate that the FDA does not consider the products to be equivalent.

The second letter of the code typically indicates the dosage form (for example, a code of AT would indicate that two topical products are equivalent).

Products with known or potential equivalency issues, but for which adequate scientific evidence exists to establish bioequivalence, are given a code of AB.

89 – a, b, d

DEA registration is not required for an agent or employee of any registered manufacturer, distributor, or dispenser if acting in the usual course of business. This includes pharmacists working at pharmacies and nurses working in a hospital or physician's office. Patients who possess controlled substances for a lawful purpose are not required to register with the DEA.

Providers must register with the DEA unless practicing under the registration of a hospital or other institution. Each pharmacy must have its own DEA registration to dispense controlled substances.

90 – d

A product is considered adulterated if its strength or quality differs from what it represents (this is not the only criteria for adulteration, but one example). A product is misbranded if the labeling is false or misleading. If a drug product's strength is less than what is represented on the label, then the drug product is considered both adulterated and misbranded.

91 – d

Patients may request easy-open containers (containers that are not child-resistant) for any prescription. A provider may also make this request on a patient's behalf (written or verbal), but can only do so for one individual prescription. Only a patient can issue a blanket request for easy-open containers on all future prescriptions. There is not a legal requirement for documentation of easy-open container requests, but it is good practice for a pharmacist to have documentation in case an issue arises.

92 – c

Risk Evaluation and Mitigation Strategies (REMS) are strategies to manage a known or potential serious risk associated with a drug. A REMS program does not have anything to do with the affordability of drugs.

93 – c

Federal regulations require a warning statement, including a warning about the risk of Reye's syndrome in children, on aspirin and other salicylate products. An example warning statement is: "Keep out of reach of children. In case of overdose, get medical help or contact a Poison Control Center right away." Containers of chewable 81mg (1.25 grain) aspirin may not contain more than 36 tablets in order to reduce the risk of accidental poisoning in children. In other words, if a child were to open a bottle of aspirin and ingest all 36 tablets, 36 tablets would generally be considered a non-toxic amount.

94 – b

DEA registration numbers begin with two letters. The first letter indicates practitioner status, in which "M" is the designation for mid-level practitioners. The second letter typically indicates the first letter of the practitioner's last name, the first letter of the pharmacy name, or the first letter of the hospital name.

To verify the DEA registration number, first add together the 1st, 3rd, and 5th digit. Then add together the 2nd, 4th, and 6th digit, and multiply this number by two. Add these two numbers together. The last digit (in the ones place) of the sum of these two numbers should match the last number of the DEA registration number.

Check each of the five choices. For the second choice (MT1200980):

1) $1 + 0 + 9 = 10$

2) $2 + 0 + 8 = 10$; $10 \times 2 = 20$

3) $10 + 20 = 30$

The last digit of 30 is 0, so 0 must be the last digit of the DEA number: MT1200980.

95 – a, b, d

The FDA requires medication guides be issued with certain prescription drugs and biologics if they determine the drug has serious risks relative to benefits, when patient adherence is crucial to the effectiveness of the drug, when there is a known serious side effect, and when providing information can prevent serious adverse effects. Medication guides do not replace pharmacist counseling. A patient also does not need to be in a nursing home to receive a medication guide. Some drugs which require a guide be dispensed with each fill are: aripiprazole, amphetamine/dextroamphetamine, fentanyl, testosterone, citalopram, ciprofloxacin, amiodarone, duloxetine, adalimumab, and more.

96 – e

Omnibus Budget Reconciliation Act of 1990 (commonly known as OBRA 90) set the requirement that patients must be offered counseling on medications. Patients have the right to refuse this counseling, but counseling must at least be offered.

97 – a, b, e

Several drugs are exempt from the child-resistant container packaging requirement. Some examples include sublingual nitroglycerin tablets, methylprednisolone tablets containing no more than 84mg per package, preparations in aerosol containers intended for inhalation, and more. Effervescent aspirin or acetaminophen tablets are exempt, but non-effervescent tablets are not. Packages of prednisone tablets are only exempt if they contain less than 105mg per package.

98 – b

Prescription records are required to be kept for a minimum of 2 years based on federal law. However, if there are stricter state laws, those should be followed. For example, if a state requires prescription records to be maintained for 5 years, then prescription records must be maintained for at least 5 years because it is stricter than 2 years.

99 – b

Aripiprazole (Abilify) is a drug that has a medication guide. Drugs that pose a serious or significant concern have medication guides. The medication guide is required for each dispensing, including refills. The medication guide is required as part of the labeling. If the medication guide is not given, the drug is considered misbranded.

100 – b

CMS regulations require a consultant pharmacist to perform a drug regimen review for long-term care patients at least once a month.

Answer Index – Tennessee Questions

1 – b, e

Federal law states that a pharmacy must notify their local DEA office in writing within one business day of discovery of significant theft or loss. In addition, the pharmacy must complete and submit DEA form 106 regarding the theft or loss.

In Tennessee, the pharmacy must report to the Board any robbery, embezzlement, theft, burglary, fire or disaster resulting in a loss of prescription drugs, controlled substances, medical devices or related materials. The report must include a list of all items and the amounts that were lost or damaged.

2 – b

The person who is taking possession of more than a seven (7) day supply of the following Schedule II–IV medications must either have identification or be known to the pharmacy staff:

- Opioids

- Benzodiazepines

- Zolpidem

- Barbiturates

- Carisoprodol

Government-issued identification or an insurance card can serve as the patient identification. If the person picking up the prescription is homeless or a minor without valid identification, the pharmacy staff may use professional judgement in determining whether to dispense the prescription to the patient.

Eszopiclone (Lunesta) is a Schedule IV hypnotic used for insomnia, like zolpidem (Ambien), but is not included in the regulation.

3 – e
The pharmacy technician to pharmacist ratio is 6:1, meaning one pharmacist can only supervise six technicians at a time. This ratio may be removed if the additional technicians are certified.

The pharmacist in charge may request a modification of the ratio from the Board of Pharmacy in writing. The pharmacist in charge must address:

- The pharmacy technician's experience, skill, knowledge and training

- The workload at the practice site

- Detailed information regarding the numbers of pharmacy technicians and the specific duties and responsibilities of each of the pharmacy technicians

- Justification that patient safety and quality of pharmacy services and care can be maintained at the pharmacy

4 – a
A prescription for a controlled substance may be partially filled if:

- The partial fill is requested by the patient or the practitioner who wrote the prescription

- The total quantity dispensed through partial fills does not exceed the total quantity prescribed for the original prescription

If a partial fill is made, the pharmacist must retain the original prescription at the pharmacy where the prescription was first presented and the partial fill dispensed. Any subsequent fill must occur at the pharmacy that initially dispensed the partial fill. Any subsequent fill must be filled within six (6) months from issuance of the original prescription, unless federal law requires it to be filled within a shorter timeframe.

If a partial fill is dispensed, the pharmacist must only record in the controlled substance database the partial fill amount actually dispensed.

When a partial fill is dispensed, the pharmacist shall notify the prescribing practitioner by one of the following:

- Through a notation in the interoperable electronic health record of the patient

- Through submission of information to the controlled substance database

- By electronic or facsimile transmission

- Through a notation in the patient's record that is maintained by the pharmacy, and that is accessible to the practitioner upon request

5 – b, c, d, e

All care and services offered under a collaborative care agreement between a pharmacy and an authorized physician, nurse practitioner or physician assistant must be pursuant of a diagnosis that was made and documented for a patient except in cases of immunizations, opioid antagonists, or preventative care. The Tennessee Board of Pharmacy provides an extensive list of what is deemed as preventative care for a patient, though it is not all inclusive. Smoking cessation and treatment of lice are both considered to be preventative care. In addition, pharmacists have no controlled drug prescriptive authority under a collaborative agreement.

6 – d

A prescription for a Schedule II controlled substance may normally be transmitted by the practitioner or the practitioner's agent to a pharmacy via fax, provided the original written and signed prescription is presented to the pharmacist for review before the dispensing of the controlled substance. Under federal law there are three exceptions in which the fax can serve as the original:

- A Schedule II narcotic to be compounded for direct patient administration via parenteral, intravenous, intramuscular, subcutaneous, or intra-spinal infusion route

- A Schedule II narcotic for a patient under hospice care (state or federal program)

- Any Schedule II substance for a resident of a long-term care facility

Tennessee closely follows federal law. The faxed prescription must be legible and transmitted by the prescriber or prescriber's agent.

A new Tennessee provision passed and implemented January 1st, 2020, states prescriptions for Schedule II drugs must be transmitted electronically with some exceptions. Additionally, a pharmacist who receives a written, oral, or faxed prescription is not required to verify with the prescriber that the prescription falls under such exceptions.

Thus, pharmacists may continue to dispense medications from valid written, oral, or faxed prescriptions.

7 – a, d

Chlordiazepoxide (Librium) is a Schedule IV benzodiazepine. Schedule III or IV drugs cannot be filled more than six (6) months from the date they were ordered by the prescriber and are not to be refilled more than five (5) times unless a new prescription is ordered by the prescriber. Additionally, any prescription for an opioid or benzodiazepine can only be dispensed in quantities of thirty (30) day supplies or less.

The person taking possession of more than a seven (7) day supply of the following Schedule II–IV drugs must have identification or be known to the pharmacy staff:

- Opioids

- Benzodiazepines

- Zolpidem

- Barbiturates

- Carisoprodol

Government-issued identification or an insurance card can serve as the patient identification. If the person picking up the prescription is homeless or a minor without valid identification, the pharmacy staff may use professional judgement in determining whether to dispense to the prescription to the patient.

Prior to prescribing more than a three-day supply of an *opioid* or an opioid dosage that exceeds a total of a one hundred eighty (180) morphine milligram equivalent dose to a woman of childbearing age (15 to 44 years of age) the prescriber must:

- Advise the patient of the risk associated with opioid use during pregnancy

- Counsel the patient on appropriate and effective forms of birth control

- Offer information about the availability of free or reduced cost birth control to the patient

These measures do not apply if the prescriber has done so in the past three (3) months or does not believe the patient is capable of becoming pregnant during the course of treatment.

8 – a

Prescription drugs and devices repackaged and used within an institution must be labeled to include:

- The name, strength, and quantity of prescription drug, device or related material, if larger than one (1), in the container

- The manufacturer's name and lot or control number

- The expiration date of the prescription drug or device or related material being repackaged

- Cautionary notations (refrigerate, shake well, not for injection), if applicable

A batch number may be assigned to products and placed on the label in lieu of the manufacturer's name and lot number. The batch number and associated manufacturer name and lot number must be recorded, maintained and readily retrievable by the pharmacy.

9 – b

Instruments or devices intended for the injection of any substance through the skin (syringes) can only be sold without a prescription if there is a proven medical need. This does not necessarily mean there must be a prescription on file to warrant proof, but the pharmacist must use professional judgment when assessing the situation. In addition, syringes must be stored in an area not accessible to the public (behind the counter).

Tennessee has adopted programs that address the use of clean needles for illicit intravenous drug use. Low cost and free syringes are available through local programs and health departments.

10 – a

The following procedures must be followed when using an automated dispensing device for storage and dispensing of capsules or tablets:

- The lot number of each drug contained must be listed or posted on the device.

- After each lot number is used the portion of the device housing the drug must be cleaned prior to refilling.

- Lot numbers may not be mixed.

- The device may be loaded by a pharmacist or a pharmacy intern/technician under the supervision of a pharmacist.

11 – c

Each pharmacy must have a current edition of the Tennessee Pharmacy Laws issued by the Tennessee Board of Pharmacy printed or electronically available in the pharmacy. In addition, an "adequate library" of references consistent with the scope of practice of the pharmacy is to be maintained. This may include material pertaining to technical, clinical and professional components of the practice of pharmacy emphasizing the specialties of the pharmacy.

12 – a, b

A prescriber treating a patient with more than sixteen (16) milligrams or equivalent of buprenorphine daily for more than thirty (30) consecutive days must clearly document in the patient record why the patient needs a higher dosage.

A prescriber treating a patient with more than twenty (20) milligrams or equivalent of buprenorphine daily for more than thirty (30) consecutive days must make an effort to consult with, or refer the patient to, an addiction specialist. If the prescriber is unable to consult with an addiction specialist, or refer the patient, then the reasons for this must be documented in the patient record.

13 – a

Each prescription must be maintained as to be readily retrieved from the pharmacy site for two (2) years from the date it was last dispensed. Prescriptions must be serially numbered and filed numerically unless administered to inpatients of an institution.

14 – c

A licensed pharmacist must complete thirty (30) hours of continuing education during each two (2) year licensing cycle. Fifteen (15) hours of continuing education must come from live contact hours. Programs can be designated "live" by an ACPE-approved provider or the Board. Pharmacists enrolled in a recognized academic program for all or part of a two (2) year licensing cycle are not required to complete continuing education. Recognized programs must be advanced or graduate level degrees in a health-related science including:

- Pharmacy

- Doctor of Medicine

- Doctor of Osteopathic Medicine

- Doctor of Dental Surgery

- Pharmacy Residency or Fellowship

- Nurse Practitioner

- Physician Assistant

15 – b, e
The immediate container of a radioactive drug must be labeled with:

- The standard radiation symbol

- The words "Caution – Radioactive Material"

- The name of the drug

- The medical or prescription order number

In addition, the immediate *outer* container must be labeled with:

- The amount of radioactive material contained

- The words "Caution – Radioactive Material"

- The radionuclide

- The chemical form

- The amount of radioactive material contained, in millicuries or microcuries

- The volume, if liquid

- The calibration time for the amount of radioactivity contained

- The expiration time

- The name, address and telephone number of the nuclear practice site.

16 – c
Gabapentin (Neurontin) is a Schedule V controlled substance in Tennessee and many other states but is not deemed a controlled substance by federal law.

Alprazolam (Xanax), carisoprodol (Soma), tramadol (Ultram) and zolpidem (Ambien) are Schedule IV controlled substances in Tennessee and federally.

17 – a, b, e

As a condition for licensure, the central pharmacy participating in the telepharmacy program must continue to meet all of the standards established in Tennessee State Pharmacy Law while also meeting the following minimum requirements:

- Maintain connection with the satellite clinic through computer, videolink and audiolink. Any interruption in connection with the satellite clinic should result in a cease of all operations in the clinic

- Ensure that prescriptions for Schedule I–IV drugs are not issued from the satellite clinic

- Ensure entry into the pharmacy (keys, etc.) is only granted to pharmacists and pharmacy technicians employed at the satellite clinic

- Proper and separate storage of drugs at the central pharmacy and satellite clinic

- Supervision of pharmacy technicians at the satellite clinic by a pharmacist without a pharmacist being physically present

- Ability to counsel patients and caregivers at the satellite clinic by telepharmacy

Clonazepam (Klonopin) is a Schedule IV benzodiazepine and hydrocodone–APAP (Norco) is a Schedule II opioid. Neither would be permitted to be issued from a satellite clinic.

18 – e

If a patient doesn't know, doesn't have or refuses to provide a social security number to enter into the controlled substance monitoring database (CSMD) the patient's driver's license number or telephone number may be used.

Furthermore, if the patient does not have a driver's license or telephone number then "000-00-0000" may be used as the patient identifier. If the patient *refuses* to provide a driver's license or telephone number then "999-99-9999" may be used as the patient identifier.

Another individual's information can all be used in the following circumstances:

- If a patient's social security number is not available, then the social security number, driver's license number or telephone number of the person obtaining the controlled substance on behalf of the patient shall be used as the patient identifier in the database or the numbers.

- If a patient is a child who does not have a social security number, then the parent's or guardian's social security number, driver's license number, or telephone number shall be used.

- If a patient is an animal, then the board shall use the owner's social security, driver's license, or telephone number.

19 – a, c, e

Wegovy (semaglutide), Phentermine, and Saxenda (liraglutide) are approved for weight loss treatment. Wegovy and Saxenda are GLP-1 receptor agonists for chronic weight management in patients with obesity or overweight conditions, while Phentermine is an appetite suppressant for short-term obesity treatment. Dexedrine and Methylphenidate are stimulants approved only for ADHD and narcolepsy, not weight loss.

20 – c

In instances where a patient's epilepsy or seizures are currently being controlled on a specific drug, strength, dosage form, and dosing regimen from a specific manufacturer, the pharmacist, pharmacist intern or technician must notify the patient (or family member, relative or friend) of any change in manufacturer. This includes interchange for:

- Generic to brand

- Brand to generic

- Generic to generic (with differing manufacturers)

The prescriber of the medication must also be notified prior to the interchange.

21 – e

A home care kit is a kit containing Board-determined drugs and is kept in the home of a home healthcare patient. The drugs are intended to be used by a healthcare professional in emergency situations. Removal of any drug must be pursuant of a prescription order or standing protocol and documented in the patient's file. When the home care kit is opened for any reason, the issuing pharmacy must be notified and then restock and reseal the home care kit in a reasonable amount of time.

The home care kit may contain:

- Sodium Chloride for Injection 0.9% Bacteriostatic

- Sterile Water for injection Bacteriostatic or Preservative Free

- Epinephrine injection 1mg/ml

- Diphenhydramine

- Heparin Flush < or = 100 units/ml

- Naloxone

- Sodium Chloride for Irrigation

- Sterile Water for Irrigation

- Dextrose 50%

- Urokinase 5000units

- Any other legend drug as approved by the board.

22 – b, d
Prescription orders for opioids and benzodiazepines may not be dispensed for quantities greater than a thirty (30) day supply.

23 – c
All drugs, devices or related materials returned to the practice site must be destroyed unless in unit dose packaging or unopened commercially prepackaged containers. In addition, the pharmacist must use professional judgment that the product continues to meet federal and state standards of integrity. For example, if a patient returns an unopened box of insulin, there is no way for the pharmacist to verify the product has been stored properly and thus should be destroyed.

24 – d
Tennessee follows federal Medicaid and Medicare requirements for tamper resistant prescriptions. To be considered tamper resistant the prescription blank must contain at the following features:

- One or more industry-recognized features designed to prevent unauthorized copying of a completed or blank prescription form

- One or more industry-recognized features designed to prevent the erasure or modification of information written on the prescription pad by the prescriber

- One or more industry-recognized features designed to prevent the use of counterfeit prescription forms.

A unique serial number may be added to the prescription blank for the purpose of tracking and enforcing potential fraud but is not mandatory. The practitioner is required to utilize reasonable safeguards to assure against theft and unauthorized use of prescriptions.

In Tennessee, a pharmacist cannot fill a prescription from a Tennessee practitioner unless it meets requirements of a tamper resistant prescription. This requirement does not apply to the following cases:

- Verbal, faxed or electronic prescription orders

- Prescription orders written by out of state practitioners

- Prescription orders written by veterinarians

- Prescription orders written for inpatient use at a hospital, nursing home, assisted living facility, mental health facility or correction facility where the order is sent directly to a pharmacy and the patient never handles the written order.

25 – b

In instances where a patient's epilepsy or seizures are currently being controlled on a specific drug, strength, dosage form, and dosing regimen from a specific manufacturer, the pharmacist, pharmacist intern or technician must notify the prescriber in addition to the patient (or family member, relative or friend) of any change in manufacturer. This includes interchange for:

- Generic to brand

- Brand to generic

- Generic to generic (with differing manufacturers)

26 – a, e

Tennessee law has set forth provisions for dispensing of new prescription orders and refills in the event of the signing prescriber's death. A new prescription order that has never been previously dispensed may be dispensed within ninety (90) days of the prescriber's death. Refills for non-controlled drugs may be dispensed within one hundred eighty (180) days of the prescriber's death. The dispensing pharmacist would have to have the knowledge of the prescriber's death and use their own professional judgement when assessing appropriateness of treatment.

The provision also mentions the refill of controlled drugs within ninety (90) days of a prescriber's death. The provision does not distinguish between controlled and non-controlled drugs as it relates to dispensing new prescription orders within ninety (90) days of a prescriber's death. Federal law is more stringent and does not allow the dispensing of a controlled substance after the death of the prescriber (DEA registration is terminated after: death, ceasing to legally exist, or discontinuation of professional practice).

The Tennessee law was enacted with the hope that federal regulation would change and there would be no further action required to implement State rules.

27 – e

A policy and procedure manual related to sterile product compounding must be available for inspection at the pharmacy practice site. The manual shall include policies and procedures for sterile compounding pursuant to USP standards, and shall, at a minimum, include:

- Security

- Equipment

- Sanitation

- Reference materials

- Prescription drug and device and related material storage

- Prescription drug and device and related material compounding and dispensing

- Prescription drug and device and related material labeling and relabeling

- Prescription drug and device and related material destruction and returns

- Dispensing of sterile products

- Record keeping

- Quality assurance

- Quality control

- Duties for pharmacist(s), pharmacy intern(s), pharmacy technician(s) and supportive personnel

- Public safety relative to harmful sterile products, including the active notification of patients if they may be affected by a product found to have a defect or an out-ofspecification result including any recall policy and procedures

- Attire

- Pharmacist, pharmacy intern, and pharmacy technician training

- Compliance with all applicable USP standards

- Response to adverse events, outbreaks, and other public health threats associated with products compounded, dispensed, manufactured, propagated, distributed, or otherwise processed at the facility, including procedures for the rapid compilation and dissemination of records to appropriate authorities

Any licensed facility which engages in sterile compounding must conduct an annual review of its policy and procedure manual, and shall update its policy and procedure manual as necessary.

28 – c
The designated pharmacist in charge (PIC) must report to the board any situation in which a medical or prescription order has caused serious personal injury or death.

The pharmacist in charge can only serve as the PIC for one pharmacy unless it is approved by the Board. The PIC must work at the pharmacy practice site 50% of hours the pharmacy is in operation but is not required to work more than forty (40) hours per week. The PIC must conduct and maintain controlled substance inventory every two years. The inventory record must include:

- The name and address of the pharmacy practice site

- The name, strength, dosage form, and quantity of each controlled substance on hand

- The date of inventory

- Whether the inventory was taken as of the opening or closing of business on that date

All other pharmacists are not relieved of their own responsibility to comply with state laws and regulations.

29 – e
When selling over-the-counter products that contain dextromethorphan, the pharmacy (or seller) must require identification to verify the buyer is eighteen (18) years of age or

Answer Index – Tennessee Questions   99 older, unless from the purchaser's outward appearance the seller would reasonably believe the purchaser to be thirty (30) years of age or older. The buyer may purchase the product if they are less than eighteen (18) years of age but must have proof of legal emancipation.

The provisions do not apply to dispensing prescription orders for products that contain dextromethorphan.

30 – a, b, d

All healthcare practitioners are required to check before dispensing an opioid or benzodiazepine as a new episode of treatment to a human patient the first time at that practice site and every 6 months thereafter when said controlled substance remains a part of the treatment for that human patient after the initial dispensing.

Healthcare practitioners are not required to check the database before prescribing or dispensing opioids or benzodiazepines if one or more of the following conditions are met:

- The controlled substance is prescribed or dispensed for a patient who is currently receiving hospice care

- The quantity of the controlled substance which is prescribed or dispensed does not exceed an amount which is adequate for a single, three-day treatment period and does not allow a refill

- The controlled substance is prescribed for administration directly to a patient during the course of inpatient or residential treatment in a hospital or nursing home licensed under title 68

31 – a, c, d

Prior to prescribing more than a three-day supply of an opioid or an opioid dosage that exceeds a total of a one hundred eighty (180) morphine milligram equivalent dose to a woman of childbearing age (15 to 44 years of age) the prescriber must:

- Advise the patient of the risk associated with opioid use during pregnancy

- Counsel the patient on appropriate and effective forms of birth control

- Offer information about the availability of free or reduced cost birth control to the patient

These measures do not apply if the prescriber has done so in the past three (3) months or does not believe the patient is capable of becoming pregnant during the course of treatment.

32 – a

Prescription drugs in an emergency room that are to be dispensed for outpatient use (other than by pharmacy staff) must be dispensed by the physician or an emergency room nurse or certified physician assistant at the direction of a physician. If the physician in an emergency room does not personally dispense, then prescription drugs for outpatient use must be packaged in containers from the pharmacy practice site in amounts not to exceed a twelve (12) hour period. Products commercially prepared for multiple dose therapy must be issued in the smallest available package size. (i.e. ophthalmic, topical and otic products). A prescription order must be issued and recorded in the emergency room and the products must be labeled with appropriate labeling.

33 – a, b, e

The dispensing label for a medical or prescription order must contain at least the following information:

- Name, address and telephone number of the pharmacy

- Medical or prescription order serial number (Rx number)

- Name of prescriber

- Name of patient

- Directions for use

- Date medical or prescription order originally dispensed and/or refill date

- Appropriate advisory label "poison", "shake", "caution"

- Name of product (unless otherwise required by the prescriber)

- Expiration date of the product (if applicable)

This rule does not apply to prescription orders dispensed by a long-term care or institution for inpatient administration.

34 – a

As a condition for licensure, the central pharmacy participating in the telepharmacy program must continue to meet all of the standards established in Tennessee State Pharmacy Law while also meeting the following minimum requirements:

- Maintaining connection with satellite clinic through computer, video link and audio link. Any interruption in connection with the satellite clinic should result in a cease of all operation in the clinic

- Ensure that prescriptions for Schedule I–IV drugs are not issued from the satellite clinic

- Ensure entry into the pharmacy (keys, etc.) is only granted to pharmacists and pharmacy technicians employed at the satellite clinic

- Proper and separate storage of drugs at the central pharmacy and satellite clinic

- Supervision of pharmacy technicians at the satellite clinic by a pharmacist without a pharmacist being physically present

- Ability to counsel patients and caregivers at the satellite clinic by telepharmacy

35 – a

Under no circumstances can a nurse practitioner or a physician assistant working under a physician's supervision be given any authority to prescribe drugs when the sole purpose is to cause or perform an abortion, including the following:

- The writing or signing a prescription for any drug or medication

- The dispensing or administration of any prescribed or legend drug or medication

- The performing of any procedure that involves the use of a legend drug or medication

36 – c

When a pharmacy initially dispenses a medical or prescription order the pharmacist must record on that prescription order:

- The date dispensed

- The pharmacist's initials

- The amount of product dispensed

If the full-face amount of the medical or prescription order is dispensed the pharmacist may date and initial the order and it is assumed that the entire amount was dispensed.

37 – c

Terms of appointment are for seven (7) years, or until their successors have been qualified, and no member of the Board is eligible for reappointment after serving a full term.

38 – a, d, e

In Tennessee, controlled substances included in Schedule VI are:

- Marijuana

- Tetrahydrocannabinol (THC)

- Synthetic equivalents of the substances contained in the plant, or in the resinous extractives of *Cannabis* sp. and/or synthetic substances, derivatives, and their isomers with similar chemical structure and pharmacological activity, such as the following:

    o 1 cis or trans tetrahydrocannabinol, and its optical isomers

    o 6 cis or trans tetrahydrocannabinol, and its optical isomers

    o 3, 4 cis or trans tetrahydrocannabinol, and its optical isomers

This does not include hemp or hemp products that meet State requirements of THC concentrations that do not exceed three-tenths of one percent (0.3%) of dry weight.

39 – a, d, e

A new Tennessee provision passed and implemented January 1st, 2020, states prescriptions for Schedule II drugs must be transmitted electronically with some exceptions. Additionally, a pharmacist who receives a written, oral, or faxed prescription is not required to verify with the prescriber that the prescription falls under such exceptions. Exceptions include:

- Issued by veterinarians

- Issued in circumstances where electronic prescribing is not available due to technological or electrical failure

- Issued by a healthcare prescriber to be dispensed by a pharmacy located outside the state, as set forth in rule

- Issued when the healthcare prescriber and dispenser are the same entity

- Issued while including elements that are not supported by the most recently implemented version of the National Council for Prescription Drug Programs Prescriber/Pharmacist Interface SCRIPT Standard

- Issued by a healthcare prescriber for a drug that the federal food and drug administration (FDA) requires the prescription to contain certain elements that are not able to be accomplished with electronic prescribing

- Issued by a healthcare prescriber allowing for the dispensing of a non-patient-specific prescription pursuant to a standing order, approved protocol for drug therapy, collaborative pharmacy practice agreement in response to a public health emergency, or in other circumstances where the healthcare prescriber may issue a non-patient-specific prescription

- Issued by a healthcare prescriber prescribing a drug under a research protocol

- Issued by a healthcare prescriber who has received a waiver or a renewed waiver for a specified period determined by the commissioner of health, not to exceed one year without renewal by the commissioner, from the requirement to use electronic prescribing, pursuant to a process established in rule by the commissioner, due to economic hardship, technological limitations that are not reasonably within the control of the healthcare prescriber, or other exceptional circumstance demonstrated by the healthcare prescriber

- Issued by a healthcare prescriber under circumstances where, notwithstanding the healthcare prescriber's present ability to make an electronic prescription as required by this subsection (a), the healthcare prescriber reasonably determines that it would be impractical for the patient to obtain substances prescribed by electronic prescription in a timely manner, and such delay would adversely impact the patient's medical condition

- Issued by a healthcare prescriber who issues fifty (50) or fewer prescriptions for Schedule II controlled substances per year

40 – d
The PIC must conduct and maintain controlled substance inventory every two years. The inventory record must include:

- The name and address of the pharmacy practice site

- The name, strength, dosage form, and quantity of each controlled substance on hand

- The date of inventory

- Whether the inventory was taken as of the opening or close of business on that date

41 – b

All licenses and certificates of registration granted by the board are for a two (2) year period beginning on the date the license is initially granted. All licenses and certificates of registration shall be renewed on or before the last day of the two (2) year license cycle. A pharmacist or pharmacy technician serving in the uniformed services of the United States is not required to pay license or registration renewal fees during the period of active duty and the pharmacist is not required to complete continuing pharmacy education requirements during the period of active duty.

42 – a, b, e

The person taking possession of more than a seven (7) day supply of the following Schedule II–IV drugs must have identification or be known to the pharmacy staff:

- Opioids

- Benzodiazepines

- Zolpidem

- Barbiturates

- Carisoprodol

Government-issued identification or an insurance card can serve as the patient identification. If the person picking up the prescription is homeless or a minor without valid identification, the pharmacy staff may use professional judgement in determining whether to dispense to the prescription to the patient.

While Tennessee law does include zolpidem (Ambien), a Schedule IV hypnotic, and carisoprodol (Soma), a Schedule IV muscle relaxant, in its requirements, not all Scheduled hypnotics or muscle relaxants are included.

43 – e

A prescriber treating a patient with more than sixteen (16) mg or equivalent of buprenorphine daily for more than thirty (30) consecutive days must clearly document in the patient record why the patient needs a higher dosage.

A prescriber treating a patient with more than twenty (20) mg or equivalent of buprenorphine daily for more than thirty (30) consecutive days must make an effort to consult with or refer the patient to an addiction specialist. If the prescriber is unable to consult with an addiction specialist or refer the patient, the reasoning must be documented in the patient record.

44 – a, c, d, e

In Tennessee, a pharmacist cannot fill a prescription from a Tennessee practitioner unless it meets requirements of a tamper resistant prescription. This requirement does not apply to the following cases:

- Verbal, faxed or electronic prescription orders

- Prescription orders written by out of state practitioners

- Prescription orders written by veterinarians

- Prescription orders written for inpatient use at a hospital, nursing home, assisted living facility, mental health facility or correction facility where the order is sent directly to a pharmacy and the patient never handles the written order

Tennessee follows federal Medicaid and Medicare requirements for tamper resistant prescriptions. To be considered tamper resistant the prescription blank must contain all the following features:

- One or more industry-recognized features designed to prevent unauthorized copying of a completed or blank prescription form

- One or more industry-recognized features designed to prevent the erasure or modification of information written on the prescription pad by the prescriber

- One or more industry-recognized features designed to prevent the use of counterfeit prescription forms.

A unique serial number may be added to the prescription blank for the purpose of tracking and enforcing potential fraud but is not mandatory. The practitioner is required to utilize reasonable safeguards to assure against theft and unauthorized use of prescriptions.

45 – c

A prescription for a controlled substance may be partially filled if:

- The partial fill is requested by the patient or the practitioner who wrote the prescription

- The total quantity dispensed through partial fills does not exceed the total quantity prescribed for the original prescription

If a partial fill is made, the pharmacist must retain the original prescription at the pharmacy where the prescription was first presented and the partial fill dispensed. Any subsequent fill must occur at the pharmacy that initially dispensed the partial fill. Any subsequent fill must be filled within six (6) months from issuance of the original prescription, unless federal law requires it to be filled within a shorter timeframe.

If a partial fill is dispensed, the pharmacist must only record in the controlled substance database the partial fill amount actually dispensed.

When a partial fill is dispensed, the pharmacist shall notify the prescribing practitioner by one of the following:

- Through a notation in the interoperable electronic health record of the patient

- Through submission of information to the controlled substance database

- By electronic or facsimile transmission

- Through a notation in the patient's record that is maintained by the pharmacy, and that is accessible to the practitioner upon request

46 – b, c

In Tennessee, the pharmacist is allowed one absence daily for up to one (1) hour. A sign containing "pharmacist not on duty" must be displayed conspicuously in the pharmacy. There must be a floor to ceiling barrier to close off the pharmacy department from the rest of the building. Prescriptions cannot be dispensed or compounded until the pharmacist returns. The pharmacist must be available to counsel patients at pick up, so prescriptions may not be sold from the will-call area either.

47 – a, b, c, d, e

Each dispenser must submit to the database all of the following information:

- Prescriber identifier

- Dispensing date of controlled substance

- Patient identifier

- Controlled substance dispensed identifier

- Quantity of controlled substance dispensed

- Strength of controlled substance dispensed

- Estimated days' supply

- Dispenser identifier

- Date the prescription was issued by the prescriber

- Whether the prescription was new or a refill

- Source of payment

- The ICD-10 code for any prescription that contains an ICD-10 code

The information in the database must be submitted for each business day but no later than the close of business on the following business day. Veterinarians must submit information at least once every 14 days and are not required to use a computerized system.

48 – b, c, e

Prescription orders for opioids and benzodiazepines may not be dispensed for quantities greater than a 30-day supply. Ativan (lorazepam) is a Schedule IV benzodiazepine while Norco (hydrocodone/APAP) and Xtampza ER (oxycodone) are Schedule II opioids.

49 – a

Tennessee law has set forth provisions for dispensing of new prescription orders and refills in the event of the signing prescriber's death. A new prescription order that has never been previously dispensed may be dispensed within ninety (90) days of the prescriber's death. Refills for non-controlled drugs may be dispensed within one hundred eighty (180) days of the prescriber's death. The dispensing pharmacist would have to have the knowledge of the prescriber's death and use their own professional judgement when assessing appropriateness of treatment. Therefore, the pharmacist does not *have* to continue refilling the prescription for this patient if it is their professional opinion that the treatment is no longer appropriate.

The provision also mentions the refill of controlled drugs within ninety (90) days of a prescriber's death. The provision does not distinguish between controlled and non-controlled drugs as it relates to dispensing new prescription orders within ninety (90) days of a prescriber's death. Federal law is more stringent and does not allow the dispensing of a controlled substance after the death of the prescriber as the DEA registration should be terminated after death, ceasing to legally exist or discontinuation of professional practice.

The Tennessee law was enacted with the hope that federal regulation would change and there would be no further action required to implement State rules.

50 – a, c, d

A home care kit is a kit containing Board-determined drugs and is kept in the home of a home healthcare patient. The drugs are intended to be used by a healthcare professional in emergency situations. Removal of any drug must be pursuant of a prescription order or standing protocol and documented in the patient's file. When the home care kit is opened for any reason, the issuing pharmacy must be notified and then restock and reseal the home care kit in a reasonable amount of time.

The home care kit may contain:

- Sodium Chloride for Injection 0.9% Bacteriostatic

- Sterile Water for injection Bacteriostatic or Preservative Free

- Epinephrine injection 1mg/ml

- Diphenhydramine

- Heparin Flush < or = 100units/ml

- Naloxone

- Sodium Chloride for Irrigation

- Sterile Water for Irrigation

- Dextrose 50%

- Urokinase 5000units

- Any other legend drug as approved by the board.

51 – e
Tennessee follows federal Medicaid requirements for tamper resistant prescriptions. To be considered tamper resistant, the prescription blank must contain the following features:

- One or more industry-recognized features designed to prevent unauthorized copying of a completed or blank prescription form

- One or more industry-recognized features designed to prevent the erasure or modification of information written on the prescription pad by the prescriber

- One or more industry-recognized features designed to prevent the use of counterfeit prescription forms

A unique serial number may be added to the prescription blank for the purpose of tracking and enforcing potential fraud but is not mandatory. The practitioner is required to utilize reasonable safeguards to assure against theft and unauthorized use of prescriptions.

In Tennessee, a pharmacist cannot fill a prescription from a Tennessee practitioner unless it meets requirements of a tamper resistant prescription. This requirement does not apply to the following cases:

- Verbal, faxed or electronic prescription orders

- Prescription orders written by out-of-state practitioners

- Prescription orders written by veterinarians

- Prescription orders written for inpatient use at a hospital, nursing home, assisted living facility, mental health facility or correction facility where the order is sent directly to a pharmacy and the patient never handles the written order.

52 – d
Copies of prescription orders issued directly to the patient by a pharmacy must have "Copy for Information Only" written in red letters that are equal in size to those describing the prescription drug. The copy does not have legal status as a valid medical or prescription order.

53 – c, d, e
When dispensing a legend drug, the label on the container must include the indication if requested by the patient, patient's caregiver or the prescriber. The indication can be provided by the patient, patient's caregiver or the prescriber.

54 – b
A pharmacist may dispense a seventy-two (72) hour supply of a non-controlled prescription if:

- The patient offers satisfactory evidence to the pharmacist that the prescriber has placed the patient on a maintenance medication and that such patient is without valid refills or for some valid reason cannot obtain proper authorization

- In the judgment of the pharmacist, the health, safety and welfare of the patient would otherwise be endangered

If proper authorization cannot be obtained during the seventy-two (72) hour period, then the pharmacist may dispense one additional seventy-two (72) hour supply to the patient.

Additionally, a pharmacist may dispense a twenty (20) day supply to patients who have been displaced by disaster and are without refills. Prescription information for these patients can be obtained from a prescription label, verbal medical order, verbal prescription order or any other means determined to be legitimate in the professional judgment of the pharmacist.

55 – d

The pharmacist must notify the patient of the substitution with a generic equivalent by noting the substitution on the prescription label. This provision does not apply to prescriptions dispensed for inpatients of a hospital, a nursing home or an assisted care living facility.

56 – d

A pharmacy that dispenses and mails a prescription into Tennessee from another state must first pay the licensure fee required of a Tennessee pharmacy. The license fees for out-of-state pharmacies and pharmacists are not to exceed those charged to Tennessee pharmacies and pharmacists.

57 – a, b, d, e

No pharmacist may dispense medication pursuant to a handwritten, typed or computer-generated prescription order unless the prescription order is comprehensible to the pharmacist.

It is the duty of the prescriber issuing the prescription order to ensure the prescription order is legible. A pharmacist must make a reasonable attempt to contact the prescriber to seek clarification of a prescription order and must not dispense the medication until clarification is obtained. Additionally, the pharmacist is not liable to any person for reasonable delay caused when seeking clarification of a prescription order.

58 – a, b, d, e

A prescription for a controlled substance may be partially filled if:

- The partial fill is requested by the patient or the practitioner who wrote the prescription

- The total quantity dispensed through partial fills does not exceed the total quantity prescribed for the original prescription.

If a partial fill is made, the pharmacist must retain the original prescription at the pharmacy where the prescription was first presented and the partial fill dispensed. Any subsequent fill must occur at the pharmacy that initially dispensed the partial fill. Any subsequent fill must be filled within six (6) months from issuance of the original prescription, unless federal law requires it to be filled within a shorter timeframe.

If a partial fill is dispensed, the pharmacist must only record in the controlled substance database the partial fill amount actually dispensed.

When a partial fill is dispensed, the pharmacist shall notify the prescribing practitioner by one of the following:

- Through a notation in the interoperable electronic health record of the patient

- Through submission of information to the controlled substance database

- By electronic or facsimile transmission

- Through a notation in the patient's record that is maintained by the pharmacy, and that is accessible to the practitioner upon request

Belsomra (suvorexant) is a Schedule IV controlled substance indicated for insomnia.

59 – d

Prior to prescribing more than a three-day supply of an opioid or an opioid dosage that exceeds a total of a one hundred eighty (180) morphine milligram equivalent dose to a woman of childbearing age (15 to 44 years of age) the prescriber must:

- Advise the patient of the risk associated with opioid use during pregnancy

- Counsel the patient on appropriate and effective forms of birth control

- Offer information about the availability of free or reduced cost birth control to the patient

These measures do not apply if the prescriber has done so in the past three (3) months or does not believe the patient is capable of becoming pregnant during the course of treatment.

60 – a, c, d

A pharmacy practice site in Tennessee must meet the following standards:

- Clean, sanitary, orderly and well-lit

- Consultation area with sufficient privacy

- Necessary counters and storage space

- Drugs, devices, apparatus and equipment sufficient to compound and dispense prescription orders

- Occupation of a space not less than one hundred eighty (180) square feet

- Hot and cold running water and immediate refrigeration

- Physical barriers for unauthorized entry

- Restriction of person(s) not practicing pharmacy

- Certificates and licenses conspicuously displayed

Additional rules apply to pharmacies located within a mercantile establishment (i.e.. grocery and department stores).

61 – c
The Board consists of 9 members to be appointed by the governor as follows: 1 consumer member; 1 registered pharmacy technician; and 7 pharmacists. The governor shall strive to ensure that at least one (1) person serving on the board is sixty (60) years of age or older, one (1) person serving on the board is a member of a racial minority, and the members on the board are representative of a variety of practice settings.

62 – e
Pharmacists, pharmacy technicians and pharmacy interns must all wear appropriate identification showing name and title.

63 – d
Patient counseling must be provided to a patient when a medical or prescription drug order is received. This includes outpatient hospitals and other institutional facilities dispensing to patients for outpatient use at discharge. There are no requirements for counseling inpatients of institutional or long-term care facilities.

64 – a, b, c, e
A pharmacist is responsible for a reasonable review of a patient's record prior to dispensing each medical or prescription order. The review must include evaluating the medical and prescription order for:

- Over-utilization or under-utilization

- Therapeutic duplication

- Drug-disease contraindication

- Drug-drug interactions

- Incorrect drug dosage or duration of drug treatment

- Drug-allergy interactions

- Clinical abuse and misuse

Upon recognizing any of the above, the pharmacist must take appropriate steps to avoid or resolve the problem.

65 – b, c, e
The Combat Methamphetamine Epidemic Act of 2005 (CMEA) sets federal purchase limits for ephedrine or pseudoephedrine base products. The daily federal limit for an authorized seller is 3.6 grams and the 30-day limit is 9 grams for retailers and 7.5 grams for mail order vendors. In Tennessee, products containing ephedrine or pseudoephedrine are limited to a more stringent 7.2 grams in any period of 30 consecutive days and 43.2 grams per year. These limits apply to a pharmacy-generated prescriptions but not prescriptions ordered from a practitioner.

66 – c
When receiving a prescription order for a drug where the prescriber did not indicate the necessity of the brand name prescribed, the pharmacist must dispense the least expensive generic equivalent in stock or the generic equivalent covered by the patient's drug plan.

67 – b, c, e
A pharmacist may provide hormonal contraceptives to a non-specific patient (over the age of eighteen (18) or otherwise legally emancipated) according to a valid collaborative agreement with a prescriber. The standardized procedures adopted by Tennessee require a pharmacist to:

- Complete a training program approved by the Department of Health related to the provision of hormonal contraceptives

- Provide the patient with a self-screening risk assessment tool developed or approved by the Department of Health

- Provide the patient with documentation about the hormonal contraceptive that was provided to the patient and advise the patient to consult with a primary care practitioner or women's healthcare practitioner

- Provide the patient with a standardized factsheet that includes, but is not limited to, the indications and contraindications for use of the drug, the appropriate method for using the drug, the importance of medical follow-up, and other appropriate information

- Provide the patient with the contact information of a primary care practitioner or women's healthcare practitioner within a reasonable period of time after provision of the hormonal contraceptive

- Either dispense the hormonal contraceptive or refer the patient to a pharmacy that may dispense the hormonal contraceptive as soon as practicable after the pharmacist determines that the patient should receive the medication.

68 – c

Unless a prescriber has specified that the dispensing the prescription with a certain initial amount with periodic refills, a pharmacist can dispense a prescription order for a non-controlled drug in varying quantities up to ninety (90) days. The dispensed quantity may not exceed the complete authorized quantity of the prescription order including refills.

69 – a

Each medical and prescription order when dispensed must be serially numbered, filed numerically and maintained so as to be readily retrievable at the pharmacy practice site for at least two (2) years from the date the medical and prescription order was last dispensed. Institutional pharmacies shall not be required to serially number medical and prescription orders dispensed for administration to inpatients of that institution.

70 – c

The pharmacist in charge (PIC) can only serve as the PIC for one pharmacy unless it is approved by the Board. The PIC must work at the pharmacy practice site 50% of hours the pharmacy is in operation but is not required to work more than forty (40) hours per week.

71 – c, d

A pharmacist or pharmacy intern, under the supervision of the pharmacist, must counsel with the person seeking to purchase a pseudoephedrine or ephedrine product and determine if it is being used for a legitimate medical purpose.

The purchaser must provide a valid government-issued photo identification and an electronic record must be maintained by the pharmacist, pharmacy technician or pharmacy intern. The electronic record must include:

- The name and address of the purchaser

- Name and quantity of product purchased

- Date and time purchased

- Purchaser identification type and number, such as driver license state and number

- The identity, such as name, initials or identification code, of the dispensing pharmacist or pharmacy intern

Beginning in 2012, this electronic information must be submitted to National Precursor Log Exchange (NPLEx). If there is a mechanical or electronic failure the pharmacy may use a written log until it is able to comply with the electronic sales tracking requirements.

72 – a, b, e

When receiving a prescription order a pharmacist must review the patient's record and personally counsel the patient or caregiver "face-to-face". If the patient or caregiver is not present, a pharmacist must then make a reasonable effort to counsel through alternative means. Alternative forms of information can be used to supplement, but not replace face-to-face counseling.

When receiving a refill for a prescription order, there must be an offer for counseling by a pharmacist, but counseling is not required unless the patient requests counseling or the pharmacist deems counseling necessary. The patient can choose to refuse counseling for any prescription order.

Patient counseling must cover matters the pharmacist deems significant including:

- The name and description of the medication

- The dosage form, dose, route of administration, and duration of drug therapy

- Special directions and precautions for preparation, administration, and use by the patient;

- Common side effects or adverse effects or interactions and therapeutic contraindications that may be encountered, including their avoidance, and the action required if they occur

- Techniques for self-monitoring drug therapy

- Proper storage

73 – e

In Tennessee, the posting of certain signage is required in healthcare provider sites. All pharmacies must have the following posted for patients:

- Contact information including the statewide toll-free number of the division of adult protective services, and the number for the local district attorney general's office

- A statement that a person of advanced age who may be the victim of abuse, neglect, or exploitation may seek assistance or file a complaint with the division concerning abuse, neglect, and exploitation

- A statement that any person, regardless of age, who may be the victim of domestic violence may call the nationwide domestic violence hotline

- A statement that a teen involved in a relationship that includes dating violence may call a national toll-free hotline

74 – a, b, c, e

A pharmacist seeking active status for an inactive, delinquent, suspended or revoked license must fulfill minimum requirements based on the time of inactivity.

If the license has been inactive, delinquent, suspended or revoked for less than one (1) year, the pharmacist must:

- Provide written notice to the board requesting an active license

- Satisfy all past due continuing pharmaceutical education as required by the board

- Pay all cumulative license renewal fees and any applicable penalty fees for the period during which the license was inactive, delinquent, suspended or revoked.

If the license has been inactive, delinquent, suspended or revoked from one (1) year to not more than five (5) consecutive years, the pharmacist must:

- Provide written notice to the board requesting an active license

- Pay all cumulative license renewal fees and any applicable penalty fees for the period during which the license was inactive, delinquent, suspended or revoked

- Satisfy all past due continuing pharmaceutical education as required by the board

- Successfully complete the jurisprudence examination

- Complete a period of pharmacy internship in Tennessee as follows:

    o If the license has been inactive, delinquent, suspended or revoked from one (1) year to not more than three (3) consecutive years, one hundred sixty (160) hours within ninety (90) consecutive days

    o If the license has been inactive, delinquent, suspended or revoked for more than three (3) consecutive years but not more than five (5) consecutive years, three hundred twenty (320) hours within one hundred eighty (180) consecutive days.

If the license has been inactive, delinquent, suspended or revoked for more than five (5) consecutive years, the pharmacist shall:

- Satisfy all past due continuing pharmaceutical education as required by the board

- Successfully complete the NAPLEX and jurisprudence examinations

- Pay all cumulative license renewal fees and any applicable penalty fees for the period during which the license was inactive, delinquent, suspended or revoked

- Complete a period of pharmacy internship of three hundred twenty (320) hours within one hundred eighty (180) consecutive days.

- Fulfill any other requirements which may be contained in any order of the board suspending or revoking the applicant's license.

Upon request, the Board may waive selected portions of these requirements.

75 – e
The person taking possession of more than a seven (7) day supply of the following Schedule II–IV drugs must have identification or be known to the pharmacy staff:

- Opioids

- Benzodiazepines

- Zolpidem

- Barbiturates

- Carisoprodol

The person taking possession of the dispensed prescription must present a valid government issued ID or public or private insurance card, unless the person is personally known to the person authorized to dispense controlled substances.

Ambien is zolpidem, Xanax is a benzodiazepine, Soma is carisoprodol, and Ultram is tramadol (an opioid). Vyvanse is lisdexamfetamine, a Schedule II stimulant for ADHD.

76 – b

The Tennessee Board of Medical Examiners adopts the following guidelines as policy for self-prescribing and for one's immediate family. For purposes of this policy, "immediate family" means a spouse, parent, child, sibling or other individual in relation to whom a physician's personal or emotional involvement may render that physician unable to exercise detached professional judgment in reaching diagnostic or therapeutic decisions. Records shall be maintained of all treatment.

Self-Prescribing:

- A physician cannot have a bona fide doctor/patient relationship with himself or herself. Therefore, except in emergency situations, a physician shall not prescribe, dispense, administer or otherwise treat himself/herself.

- Prescribing, providing, or administering of any Scheduled drug to oneself is prohibited.

Immediate Family:

- Treatment of immediate family members should be reserved only for minor, self-limited illnesses or emergency situations.

- No Scheduled drugs should be dispensed or prescribed except in emergency situations.

77 – a, b, c, e

No consumer is eligible for appointment to the Board to represent the public at large unless such person has:

- Been a resident of Tennessee for at least five (5) years

- Currently resides in Tennessee

- A non-healthcare professional by education

- No financial or other interest in any health care facility or business

78 – c

The following individuals are exempt from registration as a pharmacy technician:

- Any individual performing tasks that may be performed by a pharmacy technician who is classified by the employer as a probationary employee. The exemption shall not exceed ninety (90) days from the date of employment.

- A student enrolled in a formal pharmacy technician training program while performing experiential rotations as a part of the academic curriculum. The student shall wear a school-issued identification badge.

79 – e

A dedicated Class II type A contained vertical flow cabinet is the minimally acceptable site for compounding hazardous sterile products. Hazardous sterile products must be separated in the pharmacy practice site and storage areas must be identified.

80 – a

The pharmacy technician to pharmacist ratio is 6:1, meaning one pharmacist can only supervise six technicians at a time. This ratio may be removed if the additional technicians are certified.

The pharmacist in charge may request a modification of the ratio from the Board of Pharmacy in writing. The pharmacist in charge must address:

- The pharmacy technician's experience, skill, knowledge and training

- The workload at the practice site

- Detailed information regarding the numbers of pharmacy technicians and the specific duties and responsibilities of each of the pharmacy technicians

- Justification that patient safety and quality of pharmacy services and care can be maintained at the pharmacy.

81 – a, c, d, e

On or after January 1, 2021, any prescription for a Schedule II, III, IV, or V controlled substance issued by a prescriber who is authorized by law to prescribe the drug must be issued as an electronic prescription from the person issuing the prescription to a pharmacy. The name, address, and telephone number of the collaborating physician of an advanced practice registered nurse or physician assistant must be included on electronic prescriptions issued by an advanced practice registered nurse or physician assistant.

This does not apply to prescriptions:

- Issued by veterinarians

- Issued in circumstances where electronic prescribing is not available due to technological or electrical failure, as set forth in rule

- Issued by a health care prescriber to be dispensed by a pharmacy located outside the state, as set forth in rule

- Issued when the health care prescriber and dispenser are the same entity

- Issued while including elements that are not supported by the most recently implemented version of the National Council for Prescription Drug Programs Prescriber/Pharmacist Interface SCRIPT Standard

- Issued by a health care prescriber for a drug that the federal Food and Drug Administration (FDA) requires the prescription to contain certain elements that are not able to be accomplished with electronic prescribing

- Issued by a health care prescriber allowing for the dispensing of a non-patient-specific prescription pursuant to a standing order, approved protocol for drug therapy, collaborative pharmacy practice agreement in response to a public health emergency, or in other circumstances where the health care prescriber may issue a non-patient-specific prescription

- Issued by a health care prescriber prescribing a drug under a research protocol

- Issued by a health care prescriber who has received a waiver or a renewed waiver for a specified period determined by the commissioner of health, not to exceed one year without renewal by the commissioner, from the requirement to use electronic prescribing, pursuant to a process established in rule by the commissioner, due to economic hardship, technological limitations that are not reasonably within the control of the health care prescriber, or other exceptional circumstance demonstrated by the health care prescriber

- Issued by a health care prescriber under circumstances where, notwithstanding the health care prescriber's present ability to make an electronic prescription as required by this regulation, the health care prescriber reasonably determines that it would be impractical for the patient to obtain substances prescribed by electronic prescription in a timely manner, and such delay would adversely impact the patient's medical condition

- Issued by a health care prescriber who issues fifty (50) or fewer prescriptions for Schedule II controlled substances per year

MS Contin and hydrocodone/APAP are Schedule II controlled substances. Librium and Restoril are Schedule IV controlled substances. Repatha is not a controlled substance.

82 – b, c, d
Gabapentin ER (Horizant) is a Schedule V controlled substance in Tennessee and many other states but is not deemed a controlled substance by federal law.

Diphenoxylate/atropine (Lomotil) and pregabalin (Lyrica) are Schedule V controlled substances in Tennessee and federally.

Lorazepam (Ativan) and diazepam (Valium) are Schedule IV controlled substances in Tennessee and federally.

83 – b
A quarterly report for high risk or batch sterile products is required for all pharmacies engaged in sterile compounding unless it is a hospital pharmacy that is administering the product to inpatients or the Board has given approval. The report must be submitted by the 15th day of the month following the end of each calendar quarter. In the case of weekends and holidays the report is to be submitted on the following business day.

84 – c, d
Keys or other access devices to the physical barriers shall be subject to the following standards:

- Only pharmacists practicing at the pharmacy and pharmacists authorized by the pharmacist in charge shall be in possession of any keys or other access devices

- The pharmacist in charge shall place a key or other access device in a sealed envelope bearing the signature of the pharmacist in charge affixed across the seal and placed in a safe or vault in a secured place outside of the department. The key or access device may be used to allow emergency entrance to the department.

85 – d
No pharmacist is eligible for appointment to the Board unless such person has been a pharmacist under this or some other law of this state for a period of at least five (5) years and, during the terms of such person's incumbency, must be actively engaged in the practice of pharmacy.

86 – a, b, d, e
Each dispenser must submit to the database all of the following information:

- Prescriber identifier

- Dispensing date of controlled substance

- Patient identifier and/or client identifier

- Controlled substance dispensed identifier

- Quantity of controlled substance dispensed

- Strength of controlled substance dispensed

- Estimated number of days' supply

- Dispenser identifier

- Date the prescription was issued by the prescriber

- Whether the prescription was new or a refill

- Source of payment

Information submitted after January 1, 2016, with the exception of information reported by veterinarians, shall be submitted for each business day but no later than the close of business on the following day.

87 – e
In addition to federal requirements for DEA registration, any person that manufactures, distributes or dispenses any controlled substance must also register with the Tennessee Board of Pharmacy. All prescribers and dispensers with a DEA registration (DEA number) must also register with CSMD and comply with all reporting rules.

88 – b
At the time of dispensing of the sterile product, the dispensing container must bear a label which contains the following information:

- Patient's name (if for outpatient use) or healthcare entity name

- Prescriber (s) name (if for outpatient use)

- Pharmacy practice site name, address, and phone number (if for outpatient use)

- Identification of the pharmacist who compounded the sterile product

- When applicable, identification of the pharmacy intern or pharmacy technician who assisted in the compounding of the sterile product

- Name and amount of drug added

- Expiration date and, when applicable, expiration time, Beyond Use Dating (BUD)

- Date of compounding

- Appropriate auxiliary label(s)

- Directions for use (if for outpatient), if applicable.

89 – c

The following functions must be performed personally by a pharmacist or by a pharmacy intern under the personal supervision and in the presence of a pharmacist:

- Certification of medical and prescription orders

- Performance of final verification of the product prior to dispensing

- Initialing of medical and prescription orders noting appropriate comments

- Providing patient counseling

- Proving direct patient care services

- Providing drug information to patients, caregivers, and healthcare providers

- Supervision of compounding

- Evaluation and establishment of criteria for selection of drug product(s) and supplier(s)

- Daily opening and closing of a pharmacy practice site.

Certified pharmacy technicians may:

- Receive new or transferred oral medical and prescription orders

- Receive and transfer copies of oral medical and prescription orders between pharmacy practice sites

- Verify the contents of unit dose carts/automated dispensing systems prepared by other registered technicians when an additional verification by use of bar code technology or a licensed healthcare professional is performed prior to administration to the patient.

90 – a

Each dispenser must submit to the database all of the following information:

- Prescriber identifier

- Dispensing date of controlled substance

- Patient identifier and/or client identifier

- Controlled substance dispensed identifier

- Quantity of controlled substance dispensed

- Strength of controlled substance dispensed

- Estimated number of days' supply

- Dispenser identifier

- Date the prescription was issued by the prescriber

- Whether the prescription was new or a refill

- Source of payment

Information submitted after January 1, 2016, with the exception of information reported by veterinarians, shall be submitted for each business day but no later than the close of business on the following day.

91 – a, b, d

If a patient doesn't know, doesn't have or refuses to provide a social security number to enter into the controlled substance monitoring database (CSMD) the patient's driver's license number or telephone number may be used. Furthermore, if the patient does not have a driver's license or telephone number then "000-00-0000" may be used as the patient identifier. If the patient *refuses* to provide a driver's license or telephone number then "999-99-9999" may be used as the patient identifier.

Another individual's information can all be used in the following circumstances:

- If a patient's social security number is not available, then the social security number, driver's license number or telephone number of the person obtaining the controlled substance on behalf of the patient shall be used as the patient identifier in the database or the numbers.

- If a patient is a child who does not have a social security number, then the parent's or guardian's social security number, driver's license number, or telephone number shall be used.

- If a patient is an animal, then the board shall use the owner's social security number, driver's license number, or telephone number.

92 – b, c

Any prescription for buprenorphine monotherapy or buprenorphine without naloxone is only permitted for a patient who is:

- Pregnant

- A nursing mother

- Hypersensitive and has a documented history of an adverse reaction to naloxone

- Having the drug directly administered in the prescriber's practice site

With pregnant and nursing patients the prescriber must attempt to consult with the patient's obstetrical or gynecological provider about the appropriateness of the treatment.

93 – e

In making substitutions, the pharmacist may use drugs and drug products manufactured within the United States, or of any other country, if the products have been approved by the Food and Drug Administration (FDA), and have been given an "A" therapeutic equivalent rating by the FDA in the agency's publication, "Approved Drug Products with Therapeutic Equivalence Evaluations", also known as the "Orange Book". "A" rated drug products are those that the FDA considers to be therapeutically equivalent to other pharmaceutically equivalent products, including, but not limited to, drug products for which:

- There are no known or suspected bioequivalence problems and are designated in the Orange Book as AA, AN, AO, AP or AT.

- There are actual or potential bioequivalence problems that have been resolved with adequate in vivo or in vitro evidence supporting bioequivalence and are designated in the Orange Book as AB.

94 – a, b, c, d

At the time of dispensing of the sterile product, the dispensing container must bear a label which contains the following information:

- Patient's name (if for outpatient use) or healthcare entity name

- Prescriber's name (if for outpatient use)

- Pharmacy practice site name, address, and phone number (if for outpatient use)

- Identification of the pharmacist who compounded the sterile product

- When applicable, identification of the pharmacy intern or pharmacy technician who assisted in the compounding of the sterile product

- Name and amount of drug added

- Expiration date and, when applicable, expiration time, Beyond Use Dating (BUD)

- Date of compounding

- Appropriate auxiliary label(s)

- Directions for use (if for outpatient), if applicable.

95 – c

In addition to Schedules I–V controlled substances, Tennessee has included Schedule VI, that includes marijuana, THC and cannabis derivatives, and Schedule VII, that includes butyl nitrite ("poppers").

96 – a, c, e

Pharmacists must become licensed to practice while pharmacy technicians, certified and uncertified, must be registered. Interns and foreign graduates are not required to be licensed or registered with the Board.

97 – c

A pharmacist may dispense a seventy-two (72) hour supply of a non-controlled prescription if:

- The patient offers satisfactory evidence to the pharmacist that the prescriber has placed the patient on a maintenance medication and that such patient is without valid refills or for some valid reason cannot obtain proper authorization

- In the judgment of the pharmacist, the health, safety and welfare of the patient would otherwise be endangered

If proper authorization cannot be obtained during the seventy-two (72) hour period, then the pharmacist may dispense one (1) additional seventy-two (72) hour supply to the patient.

Additionally, a pharmacist may dispense a twenty (20) day supply to patients who have been displaced by disaster and are without refills. Prescription information for these patients can be obtained from a prescription label, verbal medical order, verbal prescription order or any other means determined to be legitimate in the professional judgment of the pharmacist.

98 – e
Butyl nitrite is used as a recreational inhalant drug commonly referred to as "poppers". Tennessee has listed butyl nitrite a Schedule VII controlled substance.

99 – c
The federally enacted Combat Methamphetamine Epidemic Act of 2005 (CMEA) sets purchase limits for ephedrine or pseudoephedrine base products. The daily limit for an authorized seller is 3.6 grams and the monthly limit is 9 grams. A mail-order or mobile vendor may only allow 7.5 grams of product to be sold every month. In Tennessee, products containing ephedrine or pseudoephedrine base are limited to a more stringent 7.2 grams in any period of 30 consecutive days and 43.2 grams per year.

Limits are calculated on the base, not salt, content of the ephedrine or pseudoephedrine in each tablet. For example, approximately 18 percent of the molecular weight of a 30 mg tablet of pseudoephedrine HCl weight is hydrochloric salt. Therefore, a 30 mg tablet of pseudoephedrine HCl has 24.6 mg of pseudoephedrine base.

7.2 grams allowed in 30-day period:

292 tablets x 24.6 mg pseudoephedrine base per tablet = 7183.2 mg = 7.1832 grams

100 – b
The chief medical officer is authorized to implement a state-wide collaborative pharmacy practice agreement specific to opioid antagonist therapy with any pharmacist licensed in, and practicing in, this state. A pharmacist licensed in, and practicing in, this state is authorized to dispense an opioid antagonist, in good faith, pursuant to a valid state-wide collaborative pharmacy practice agreement executed by the chief medical officer. Under a valid state-wide collaborative pharmacy practice agreement authorized by the chief medical officer, an authorized pharmacist may dispense an opioid antagonist to:

- A person at risk of experiencing an opiate-related overdose

- A family member, friend, or other person in a position to assist a person at risk of experiencing an opiate-related overdose

Before a pharmacist enters into a state-wide collaborative pharmacy practice agreement with the chief medical officer for the dispensing of an opioid antagonist, the pharmacist shall be able to provide documentation of completion of an opioid antagonist training program within the previous two (2) years.

The pharmacist shall maintain the collaborative pharmacy practice agreement in accordance with the requirements set forth in § 63-10-217, and this agreement must be made available to the Department of Health upon request.

A pharmacy may still dispense opioid antagonists pursuant to a valid prescription drug order.

Contact Us

Pharmacy Testing Solutions is committed to publishing high-quality, accurate test prep materials. We have had multiple pharmacists review this material as well as a copyeditor. However, despite our best efforts, we realize that an occasional error may occur. If you encounter anything that appears to be incorrect, please contact us!

We will immediately review the issue and publish a correction if necessary. This will help to ensure that our content is 100% accurate for future students. And we will also send you a nice reward for any significant errors that are brought to our attention. You may contact us at: PharmacyTestingSolutions@gmail.com.

Thanks for choosing our MPJE review book!

Made in the USA
Monee, IL
08 July 2025

20752237R00072